Jenny Brockis is an extremely knowl
and an outstanding presenter who gen
with the world in her book *Thriving*
on her own story of what many face today. That is surviving,
rather than thriving, in a VUCA (volatile, uncertain, complex and
ambiguous) world. For many others this is combined with attempts
to not only achieve but maintain high levels of performance at the
cost of wellbeing. Jenny knows her stuff and genuinely shares the
science in a palatable and honest way that readers can relate to. She's
successfully combined the science of Positive Psychology (the science
of optimal human functioning) with broader wellbeing science and
offered the reader the knowledge and skills to create a thriving life, a
good life. There's a pearl of wisdom in this book for everyone.

Dr Suzy Green, The Positivity Institute

In this book, Dr Jenny Brockis tells us gently but warmheartedly
how we can be the main character of our own lives. This is very
timely, since many of us are suffering from geopolitical events,
natural disasters and a pandemic, and looking for the new
normal. It is never too late for us to adapt and thrive to have
'happiness'. After reading the book, I felt as if today was the first
day of the rest of my life.

Professor Ken Nosaka, PhD, Director of Exercise and
Sports Science, School of Medical and Health Sciences,
Edith Cowan University

In *Thriving Mind* Dr Jenny Brockis has touched on something
so many of us experience on a daily basis. We're pushing
ourselves too hard in the relentless pursuit of success and paying
a heavy price — personally and professionally. Her pragmatic
approach based on her own experiences and depth of knowledge
is empowering and transformative, which will help us all to
become our brilliant selves — and isn't that what we all want for
our organisations, teams, ourselves and our families? A must
read for anyone wanting to thrive is today's world.

Janine Garner, best-selling author of *Be Brilliant* and
It's Who You Know, founder of LBDGroup

What a rich and wonderful tapestry of valuable information Jenny has woven with this book. She has pulled together a hundred disparate threads of wellbeing knowledge, interlaced them with research, her own story and her deep determination to help others. If you wanted just one book that brings it all together, then this would be the one. This book is packed with insight and easily accessible information on which you can take ACTION!

Isobel Colson, The Get Going Coach

This book is of, and from, the brain, heart and soul. All the things that make a whole, insightful and compassionate read from a professional who dares to be brave, vulnerable and, importantly, who shares. It is well-researched and evidence-based and is profoundly helpful and practical for all ages. I heartily recommend it!

Denise Clarke-Hundley, Community Outreach worker

In *Thriving Mind*, Dr Jenny Brockis shares her personal experience and insights, providing a variety of practical ideas for preventing overwork, burnout, lack of mental well-being, and loneliness. Drawing on the findings of science and positive psychology, she offers an easy-to-use framework for becoming a 'happy, thriving, human.' In a world overcome with challenges, uncertainty, and constant change, Dr Brockis provides comfort, optimism, and hope.

Paul and Erin Kurchina, directors, KurMeta Group

Dr Jenny Brockis is to be applauded for penning a concise, interesting and informative book. Dr Brockis has reviewed volumes of international research and synthesized it into a reader-friendly book with 'actionable' advice. From the curious reader to healthcare professionals seeking evidence-informed recommendations, *Thriving Mind* has something for everyone. Once again, Dr Brockis proves why she is a trusted authority on the links between lifestyle and vitality!

Alan C. Logan, co-Author of *Your Brain on Nature*

WOW, WOW, WOW! What a life changing book. I was more than aware of my habit of putting my career, work and business ahead of not only my health, but everything in my life, but doing something about it has been a long-standing quest. In *Thriving Mind*, Jenny not only identifies the true implications of this imbalance, but provides unbelievably straightforward and actionable steps to get that balance back. This isn't just another health book or theory, this is a game changer. If you are wondering if there is a way to feel happier and healthier while balancing big responsibilities – there is, and the answers are on these pages!

Kylie Clark, General Manager, Preacta Recruitment

When it comes to helping others to build resilience, positivity and a healthy state of mind, Dr Jenny Brockis never fails to deliver. This masterpiece arms you with all the tools needed to ensure your life journey is one that will enable you to be more balanced, mentally agile and productive. It's the very type of book you wish you had when you first set out on adulthood.

Emeritus Professor Gary Martin FAIM FACE, CEO,
Australian Institute of Management, Western Australia

Thriving Mind

Thriving Mind

HOW TO CULTIVATE A GOOD LIFE

DR JENNY BROCKIS

WILEY

First published in 2020 by John Wiley & Sons Australia, Ltd
42 McDougall St, Milton Qld 4064

Office also in Melbourne

Typeset in Warnock Pro Regular 11/14pt

© John Wiley & Sons Australia, Ltd 2020

The moral rights of the author have been asserted

ISBN: 978-0-730-38365-9

A catalogue record for this book is available from the National Library of Australia

Cover design by Wiley

Cover image © Yifei Fang / Getty Images

Printed in Singapore by Markono Print Media Pte Ltd

10 9 8 7 6 5 4 3 2 1

Disclaimer

To John
You were always born to fly

Contents

About the author   *xiii*
Acknowledgements   *xv*
Introduction   *xvii*

Part I: DISRUPTION   **1**
1 Don't panic, but dinner is burning in the oven   3
2 Reconnecting to what matters   25

Part II: HAPPINESS   **31**
3 Purpose and meaning — for a reason   39
4 Grateful for gratitude   49
5 Helping out helps everyone   57
6 Mindfully yours   65
7 Laugh and play makes your day   85
8 Mindset — dial up the positive   99

Part III: THRIVING   **113**
9   Rest and recovery — the key to resilience   117
10 Sleep — not just for the wicked   131
11 Food to boost your mood   153
12 Exercise as medicine   173
13 Music and dance   191
14 Blue and green — complete the scene   203

Part IV: HUMAN   **215**

15 Trust and respect   225
16 Kindness and compassion   243
17 Empathy: 'I feel your pain'   253

Conclusion: The times are a-changin', and so can you   *263*
A note from Jenny   *273*
References   *275*
Index   *291*

About the author

Jenny Brockis is ever curious to discover what will help others find greater happiness, better health and fulfillment in life and work.

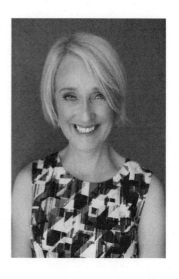

As a medical practitioner and board-certified lifestyle medicine physician she is committed to raising awareness of what the science has shown is possible. She remains optimistic we can design a better, healthier and kinder future to support ourselves and thrive, while also taking care of our beautiful and fragile planet.

She is the Founder and Director of her company Brain Fit and the author of three previous books *Brain Fit!*, *Brain Smart* and the best seller *Future Brain* (Wiley) that was released in a second edition as *Smarter Sharper Thinking*.

To learn more about her work, visit drjennybrockis.com

Acknowledgements

Saying thank you doesn't feel quite enough when trying to express my deep gratitude to everyone who helped this book come to life. But here goes because without you all, this manuscript would never have been written.

To the Wiley team who entrusted me to deliver. To Lucy Raymond senior commissioning editor, Chris Shorten and Bronwyn Evans. To my extraordinary book coach Kelly Irving, who pushed hard on getting the structure right, Lu Saxton wordsmith and editor who kept me on track and stopped me from diving down too many other rabbit holes of interest and Jem Bates for applying the final spit and polish.

To my brilliant mentor Janine Garner, fellow Yorkshire lass. Thank you for your unwavering support and ongoing supply of Big Girl Undies. To the members of Inner Circle – wow. It's such a joy to be a part of such a wonderful and inspiring group of smart, sassy female leaders. Thank you for challenging me to be the brave rebel, bucking conformity, never permitting mediocrity and sharing so much fun and laughter. Drinking chocolate will never be the same.

To my wonderful friends who don't take 'no' for an answer when inviting me out to play. Thank you for always including me even when I can't be with you because of travel commitments, and for keeping me accountable to my own wellbeing. You know who you are, and thank you.

To all the people I admire deeply for their expertise and willingness to share their thoughts for the book. Alex Kjerulf, Emiliana Simon-Thomas, Dan Diamond, Alex Logan, Susan Prescott, Ken Nosaka and to Paul Kurchina, chief cheerleader and promoter. Thank you so very much.

My thanks too, to the person to whom this book is dedicated, John. You have always kept me safe and encouraged me to grow my own wings and fly. Your sage advice given with love to 'Build Well and Fly Safe' means we'll always be flying together. And to Tom and Sophie as you continue to follow your dreams; stay happy and embrace all the possibilities of what the world has to offer. I am so proud of you both and love you to bits.

Thank you too for choosing to read this book, to be willing to explore what could be different or improved on. If you're looking to let go of what doesn't serve you well and to cultivate the success and happiness you desire to fully thrive, my hope is this book will help you achieve that.

Introduction

An ounce of prevention is worth a pound of cure.
Benjamin Franklin

Squinting into the bright sunlight as I stepped out of the Dash-8 aircraft onto the tarmac, a tingle of excitement ran through my body. We were here! A week-long break stretched out before us in which to relax, refresh and restore on the magical island of Lord Howe, off the New South Wales coast.

It had been a busy year, with work taking me to speak at conferences at a range of different destinations around Australia, New Zealand and beyond. While I love travelling, particularly to places I don't know, the long hauls especially can be tiring and the jet lag debilitating. It can often be lonely too. After a while all the hotel rooms start to look the same and eating alone, even in a nice restaurant, isn't much fun, especially when you're missing your family.

I'd had a number of personal issues to deal with as well. My dad had died at the beginning of the year and Mum, who had been his full-time carer for five years, went into a steep downward spiral mentally, cognitively and physically, until we thought we were going to lose her too before the year was out.

Taking this time out with just John, my hubby, was important for both of us. We had both been so darn busy with all our 'stuff' and needed to rejuvenate our relationship after spending so much time like ships passing in the night. Our plan was to devote this precious break to the activities we've always loved in beautiful locations — swimming, snorkelling, walking, climbing and cycling.

Best of all we were in an Internet-free zone with no mobile coverage, so we were on a digital detox! My smartphone was now relegated to being just a camera. Initially I found I kept picking it up as if to reassure myself it still worked, though all it showed was 'No service'. Clearly I'm more of an addict than I realised.

Enjoying our technology- and media-free interlude quickly led to a rapid reduction in stress levels. I couldn't remember feeling so relaxed and happy for years.

I'm sure you can relate.

Have you been hanging out for time off? Are you fed up with feeling chronically tired, sleep deprived, frustrated by your own shortcomings (and those of other people) and more than a tad anxious about what your future might hold?

It's no secret. Our world of constant and rapid change, new technologies, high expectations, economic uncertainties and geopolitical upheavals has placed a heavy weight on our shoulders and we're paying a high price for it. When we're under too much pressure it's harder to find the patience, kindness and compassion we need to flourish. We treasure the idea of changing course towards being happy and healthy, but our perpetual state of busyness means those good intentions packed their bags and left the building some time ago.

 Does it feel to you that it's getting harder to be a good human?

As a medical practitioner and lifestyle medicine physician I'm deeply concerned by the growing levels of chronic disease, poor mental health, unhappiness and loneliness in our society. Why is it that while all our cleverness has allowed us to achieve so much, we appear to be going backwards in terms of self-care, mental wellbeing and human connection?

The irony for me was that what I do gave me particular insights into just how much I needed that holiday, which is the problem for many of us. Hanging out for that weekend away, short break or scheduled time off reflects our need for more ways to ensure we can refresh and restore in our everyday life, rather than waiting until we're on the brink of exhaustion. Sustainability is the name of the game we need to play.

I wrote this book not just to share my holiday itinerary (though I'm happy to show you the pics any time), but to provide you with a guide to what you can do to increase your own happiness and wellbeing in order to truly flourish as the best human being you can be.

Think of it as a resource of reminders to help prevent you from getting caught up in the melee of overwork, burnout and poor health, because none of us are immune.

I know this to be true because I chose to wear my superhero cape for a while until, like Icarus, I flew too close to the sun and plummeted back to Earth.

When I found myself stuck in bed, unable to summon the energy to get up, let alone get dressed, it was hard to come to terms with what was happening. Waves of panic, disordered thinking and suicidal ideation blinded me to the understanding that I was simply burnt out.

The more I tried to be 'normal', the worse I felt. The more I sought to keep everything on track, the more I failed.

I didn't want to believe the reality, because hey, I was invincible. I was a superhero. Having strived hard, I had created and ran a successful group medical practice. I had two beautiful children and a loving husband who was a rock of support and unconditional love. I had it all.

 I had succeeded in achieving my goals. Isn't that what most of us aim for?

The irony of falling foul of burnout despite 'knowing' how to stay happy and healthy was not lost on me. It compounded my sense of ignominy and shame. *Call yourself a doctor? Didn't they give you the manual at medical school on how to look after yourself?*

No one chooses burnout, and it doesn't happen overnight.

For months I had ignored the tell-tale signs that I had been pushing too hard for too long. Yes, I was tired, but what did I expect? I was working full time, and the responsibilities of being a business owner meant it wasn't finished when the last patient of the day had gone and the door to the surgery closed. I had no training in the administrative demands of running a business so I had to learn as I went along, and this consumed a good deal of my down time after hours and on weekends.

Managing my staff meant I was at once a diplomat, a counsellor and a peacemaker, while at the same time inspiring the highest standard of service to match my own perfectionist tendencies. When an associate called in sick or took leave, I filled the gap.

Taking time off was tricky, and I found I was still thinking about work when away from the office. Work lost its sparkle. Having put so much of myself into creating the practice of my dreams, I now dreaded the drive to the surgery. I found it harder to be as interested in my patients and felt like a fraud.

When did I stop caring?

With little appetite for my work or food, I lost nine kilos in weight. Patients were quietly asking the receptionist, 'Is Dr Jenny all right?' Or even 'Is it cancer?'

Compounding my distress was the worst business decision I ever made. I took on a business partner who even before the ink had dried on the contract I knew to be completely incompatible with my values and beliefs around how a successful medical practice should run.

When the waves of panic started to surge, I disassociated from them. Hmm, so this is what a panic attack feels like? No worries, I know they won't kill me.

The suicidal ideation was more concerning. I started to have recurrent thoughts around the idea that my kids would be better off without me, that my husband would find greater happiness with someone not as screwed up as his current wife, and I wondered what it would be like to run my car off the road into a tree.

Distressed by these thoughts yet unwilling to admit I needed help, I kept my pain to myself.

Having looked after some of my patients who were victims of disordered thinking, I could relate to how they came to feel such a lack of self-worth.

Fortunately, something unexpected happened before my depression took too firm a hold. The smack on the head I needed to get help occurred during an appointment with a therapist, while seeking treatment for the chronic neck and shoulder pain I'd been experiencing.

I passed out.

After coming round, I gathered my thoughts and took myself home thinking, it's a long weekend, I'll be fine for Tuesday, I just need some rest.

That rest turned into what I came to call my Gap Year.

Recovery from burnout is slow. Fortunately, I had help from a wonderful and highly compassionate psychologist who wasn't afraid to ask the challenging questions. His 'And how did you contribute to the situation?' knocked me out of victimhood. My choices to put everything and everyone else before my own needs and self-care had indeed contributed to my eventual burnout.

Over the months my husband and beautiful friends continued to support my recovery.

As a doctor, perfectionist and people pleaser I felt I had let everyone down, including myself. I felt stupid. Learning self-acceptance and self-compassion was hard and remains a work in progress today.

My story of burnout, anxiety and depression is hardly unique, but shame kept me from talking openly about it. For a long time I chose not to share what had happened out of fear of being judged, of being seen as weak, incompetent, a failure.

I buried it deep.

But life has moved on and I now find myself in a new role as a workplace consultant and keynote speaker specialising in brain health, mental wellbeing and mental performance. Ever fascinated by the new findings emerging from neuroscience, behavioural science and positive psychology, the more I have delved into the research the more convinced I have become that every one of us has the capacity to adapt and thrive, and to enjoy a truly fulfilling life.

I'm sharing my story with you because no-one is immune to the consequences of poorly managed, chronic occupational stress and my hope is that reading this book may help you avoid making the same mistakes I did by knowing how to recognise the signs, and how to reduce your own risk and stay safe.

As Benjamin Franklin suggests, prevention is key.

This book is divided into four parts. In the first part, I explore the reasons why we have become at risk, how our maladaptive behaviours show up and the challenges we face to successfully adapt. In parts II, III and IV we'll look at the three components of becoming a 'happy thriving human'. It's all about:

- how to elevate your mental and emotional wellbeing in order to be HAPPIER

- how to successfully incorporate better self-care into your daily schedule to truly THRIVE

- how to harness the power of human connection to create deep and meaningful relationships and feel fully HUMAN.

In the conclusion we'll review the *what* and the *how* and *where* to go from here. Finally, I've collected some links to additional useful resources on my website.

Are you ready to give yourself permission to be the best you can be and to accept that you are *enough*? Are you willing to accept there may be certain items in your mental toolbox that don't serve you well, or as Marie Kondo would say, 'no longer give you joy'? *Let's toss them out.* Are you able to take on board and commit to adopting a more fulfilling life? Because you can be happy, healthy *and* successful.

Welcome to *Thriving Mind*. I hope you enjoy it.

Part I

Disruption

**Embracing
opportunities to change**

Somewhere, somehow there came a tipping point where despite all our cleverness and desire to forge a bright shiny future we forgot something important. The one thing that enables us to bring our best selves to everything we do. The one thing that helps us successfully navigate life's ups and downs. The thing that best prepares us for 'what's next?'

That one precious thing? That we are human; fallible, vulnerable and, as Professor Dan Ariely likes to remind us, 'predictably irrational'.

Because being human brings responsibility:

⚜ to take care of ourselves, and to maintain good physical health and mental wellbeing in order to think well, make good decisions, learn effectively and feel happy

⚜ to nurture the relationships that bind us to one another as communities, stronger bonds creating greater cohesion, collaboration and trust

⚜ to take care of the planet and our environment

⚜ to embrace activities that engage our curiosity and stretch our imagination, promoting greater creativity and innovation. Where would we be without music and dance, the arts and the inspiration nature provides?

In part I of the book I unpack some of the elements that have contributed to the rising tide of anxiety, depression, overwhelm and loneliness that are leading to greater unhappiness, poorer health and rising dissatisfaction at work.

If you are in that place where you too are worried about what the future might bring and want to be best prepared to move forward with confidence and some element of certainty, stepping back to examine where we have veered off course provides a starting point for recovery and restoration.

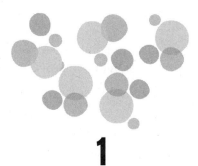

1

Don't panic, but dinner is burning in the oven

When caught up in our too-busy bubble we become blind to how
it happened and too time-poor to fix it.
J.B.

Imagine waking up every morning feeling refreshed, energised and excited for the day ahead, enjoying that quiet sense of satisfaction that all's well with the world. You're happy, healthy and thriving in your work and life.

How wonderful. But what if your reality looks a little different? Like last Tuesday.

You oversleep, so you don't have time to pick up a coffee on the way to work. Some rude jerk cuts you off in the traffic and you get into the office to face an angry colleague who blames you for some document that didn't get sent to the right person.

You've got 10 reminders on your phone telling you you're late for the monthly staff meeting, and you've just noticed that in your haste to get out of the door you blindly picked up a pair of shoes that seemed to match ... but not in colour.

All this along with the usual daily barrage of emails, phone calls, meetings, more meetings and a couple of extra meetings before you can get onto your real work. And always the undercurrent of economic uncertainty, worrying about your job security and chronic work overload. There's no time to scratch yourself let alone take a toilet break or have lunch, and you're feeling more than a little frazzled.

It's been said work is good for us but when did it become acceptable, expected even, that it's okay to dedicate your life, like a sacrificial lamb, on the high altar of work, forgoing all that makes you feel truly fulfilled and happy? How is it that in this time of golden opportunity and possibility, when we are witnessing so much positive change — from new digital technologies to advances in health care, healthy food and education — that it seems nigh on impossible to carve out enough time and energy to engage with all the multiple facets of your life that make you feel complete?

Why are so many people experiencing such high levels of stress that it's impacting their health and wellbeing? Rising levels of mental health issues and burnout are a massive problem in almost every workplace.

The new norm of constant, fast and radical change has resulted in an alarming increase in maladaptive behaviours and thinking patterns. Much of the time we're over-worrying and overthinking, pushing harder all the time to get everything done against a backdrop of chronic fatigue. Little wonder we sometimes get it wrong and end up feeling overstretched, worried and exhausted to the extent that our physical health and mental wellbeing are put at risk and the threat of burnout looms large.

Too tired to care

When overthinking becomes the norm, worrying about making a mistake, meeting deadlines, sorting out relationship conflicts and differences of opinion can weigh you down. When you're time poor, trying to clear the backlog of so many competing thoughts leads you to feeling under continual pressure. No wonder you're tired and stressed.

If you've abandoned self-care—because who's got time for that?—can you remember a different time when you used to get to the gym regularly, always caught up with your friends on a Friday night, and felt in control of your life and destiny?

It can be frustrating if you want your life to be different, better, and maybe you don't like the person you've become: tetchy, irritable and sometimes a little unkind. You may hear yourself saying things in the heat of the moment that are horrid, uncalled for and deeply wounding. Even if it wasn't your intent, you know just how damaging this can be to your relationships.

You know you're better than this, and capable of so much more. But for now you're too busy papering over the cracks, hoping others, including your boss, won't notice.

And what if you *are* the boss? Are others giving you that sideways glance, wondering why you're not delivering on the potential they previously saw in you? Were they mistaken in their estimation of and trust in you?

Most destructive is the nagging seed of self-doubt, knowing that staying on this hamster wheel without knowing how to get off means perpetuating and nurturing this monster of our own making, leading us to an uncertain and unhappy future.

It's time to take a step back to examine what got us here and what can be done to rectify the situation. Because it doesn't have to be like this.

The solution lies in recognising what's been getting in our way and knowing what to do about it, while understanding we'll find no one-size-fits-all answer. The big issues include:

- **lack of mental wellbeing**. We've lost sight of what makes us happy.

- **overwork, stress and burnout**. We're not managing our wellbeing.

- **a sense of disconnect and loneliness**. We're losing real human connection.

Let's take a look at each of these issues in turn.

Lack of mental wellbeing

Your mental wellbeing is what allows you to work to the best of your ability, to cope well with the normal stresses of everyday life, to feel productive and useful, knowing you are contributing towards something bigger than yourself. It's what makes you happy. Which is why in this increasingly complex and demanding world taking good care of your mental wellbeing matters. It keeps you safe from falling foul of mental distress and the risk of developing a mood disorder such as anxiety or depression.

How you show up each day depends on a variety of factors: how well you slept, how much you have on your mind and what's worrying you (did you remember to take the washing out of the machine to dry last night, because you wanted to wear a particular shirt today?). Juggling all these sorts of concerns on your mental to-do list is normal and something you do every day. But this is about recognising when the warning light is flashing on your mental dashboard to indicate you've reached your limit, and we all have a limit.

Avoiding the safety hazards

Identifying and avoiding the multitude of trip hazards that can put your mental wellbeing at risk is a bit like trying to navigate an obstacle course where the obstacles keep changing in size, number and position. Some feel easier to overcome than others; some rarely show up while others pop up every day as if to taunt you.

No two people share the same trip hazard list, but there may be considerable overlap when dealing with mental overload, fatigue, a toxic working environment or a difficult relationship.

It takes courage (and insight) to acknowledge that a problem exists. Reasons for ignoring your trip hazards can include:

- failing to recognise the level of your mental distress
- wanting to resolve your difficulties yourself without help
- stigmatising beliefs such as fear of judgement or being considered weak, or feelings of shame.

The danger here is that failing to get help early enough will delay diagnosis or getting extra support. Your mental wellbeing is something that requires your attention every single day, and it starts with your asking the question, *How am I feeling?*

If the answer is 'not great', then it's time to move into action to remedy the cause and get back on track towards feeling great again. The good news is, there are many strategies you can use to do this. These will be explored in part II of this book.

The agony of anxiety

One of the biggest issues many of my clients face is anxiety generated by the uncertainties of modern life. With overwhelm on pretty much everyone's CV, how do you cope when your usual stress levels just quadrupled because some of your key work colleagues are on sick leave, you've got a new client who is proving exceptionally demanding, or you've been missing out on sleep because you're worried about your parents' increasing frailty.

Then there's job insecurity. Do you worry about how long it will be before your role is replaced through artificial intelligence, automation and robotics? Another common fear is concern for the future, whether it's about climate change, geopolitical instability or the possibility of economic recession. Not having the answers to these weighty challenges can itself take a heavy toll.

Anxiety can sneak up on you if you're caught in a toxic work environment where you're afraid to speak up or to seek clarification because the prevailing culture will punish you if you're seen as being weak or incompetent. How can you deliver your best when you're unsure what's expected of you? This uncertainty can lead to procrastination and perpetuate an undercurrent of fear. You're stuck, wheels spinning, not getting anywhere fast. Anxiety, especially when accompanied by perfectionism and impostor syndrome, is our number one productivity killer, stymieing success in exams, performance reviews and career progression. Worry about not being good enough, or downplaying your achievements because you're afraid of being exposed as a fraud, is a real bummer.

Anxiety develops when your worries feel uncontrollable and relentless. If this has been happening to you for more than six months and is accompanied by difficulty concentrating, fatigue, restlessness, irritability, muscle tension or sleep disturbance, you may have an anxiety disorder.

What? You thought it was normal to feel like this? The problem is, if it's been happening for a while, it's become your normal. But it's not. Normal, that is. Which is why knowing things can be different can be hugely reassuring. Better still, you get to choose the *what*, know your *why* and, after reading the book, the *how* too.

The darkness of depression

Alongside anxiety the other saboteur of mental wellbeing is depression. Sometimes they turn up together. Depression manifests as a debilitating, unrelenting sense of deep unhappiness that is much more than a case of feeling a bit blue or having a 'bad hair day'.

A diagnosis of depression might be suggested if over the past two weeks you've experienced five or more of the following symptoms:

+ sadness or a depressed mood

+ lack of pleasure in those activities you normally enjoy

+ trouble sleeping

+ lack of energy

+ feelings of worthlessness or guilt

+ difficulty staying focused

+ a big change in appetite

+ feelings of agitation

+ suicidal ideation.

If you think this is you it's time to put your hand up and ask for help, because depression can have many contributing causes, can vary in severity and can require medication or other forms of treatment to get you back to normal.

This is the time to acknowledge that things aren't right and to call it out for what it is. You are suffering from depression. Expressing how you feel can be hard, but sharing your emotions in this way has been shown to reduce its intensity and makes it easier for family and friends to support you more effectively.

Overwork, stress and burnout

Overwork has crept into our culture like a stealth bomber. When you're loving your work, hungry to advance and keen to show your commitment to the cause, you do what's needed to show your capability, working harder than most, pulling out all the stops to ensure your success.

There's just one problem. Overwork isn't the yellow brick road to success; it's a fast track to poorer performance, stress-related illness, mental mood disorders and in extreme cases even death.

 The truth is, overwork is killing us.

Are you working too hard?

Studies have shown that the optimum length of the work week is about 38 hours; some work productivity specialists say 35 would be better. Stanford economics professor John Pencavel found that productivity drops sharply after 50 hours, and that working beyond 55 hours a week is unproductive.

Why? Because your physiology and psychology are optimised to operate at a certain level beyond which no further gains are obtained and you run the risk of blowing your head gasket. If you're consistently putting in many more hours than you're contracted for, the really disappointing news is you're not going to be any more productive than if you were working less. Which makes the pain of putting up with overwork feel even worse.

Flexible work hours with the option of working from home sounds great, but blurring the line between work and leisure hours can also contribute to that sense of always being 'on-call and contactable'.

When overwork is part of the workplace culture, you don't want to be seen as the slacker skiving off because you don't want to miss your daughter's piano recital or, heaven forbid, leaving because it's knocking-off time. When you fear that saying 'no' could compromise your job security, how do you refuse that request to stay late, again?

The health risks of overwork

In Japan they call it *karoshi*. In China it's known as *guolaosi* and in Korea *gwarosa*. It's death from overwork due to heart attack, stroke or suicide. Australia doesn't collect statistics on stress-related deaths, so it's difficult to gauge the extent of the problem in this country, but how often have you heard of someone who suffered a heart attack or stroke in which overwork was suspected to have played a role? None of us are immune to the risk.

Overwork raises levels of cortisol and adrenaline, our stress hormones. A review led by University College London analysed data from 25 studies involving more than 600 000 people and another 17 studies of 528 000 people and found that those who worked more than 11 hours a day increased their risk of heart attack by 67 per cent compared with those who worked 7–8 hours.

Compared with working a standard week of 35–40 hours, even after accounting for other risk factors such as age, sex and socioeconomic status, the review found that working more than 55 hours a week increases our risk of stroke by 33 per cent and heart attack by 13 per cent.

If overwork is your routine practice, you could end up stuck in the brown-out zone, which as the name suggests isn't the most pleasant place to be.

Brown-out is that horrible sense of being ground down by the weight of too much to do, too much responsibility and too much expectation hanging around your neck like the proverbial albatross. You know that if you are requested to please do more with less one more time you'll have an attack of the screaming heebie-jeebies.

If you're locked down in brown-out while your organisation is experiencing downsizing, a merger or organisational change, you may have noticed how those left behind are now expected to shoulder the burden, to take on extra duties and responsibilities with less backup and support. While this may be manageable in the short term, what happens when there's no Plan B for change for the foreseeable future?

Under pressure you start to cut corners, like choosing not to fact check or scrutinise your work for errors. The quality of your work starts to slide. Your decision making is impacted because you aren't applying critical thinking, and because you're always in a rush you have no time to reflect on how things are progressing, although the knot in your stomach is telling you things aren't as they should be. Sinking further into brown-out you find you've lost your 'mojo'. You're now in the first phase of burnout.

Burnout: It's the real thing

Burnout is devastating for the person affected, while the fallout also impacts their family, friends, work colleagues and the company.

And it's a growing problem.

The rising prevalence of burnout is recognised in the new edition of the WHO's International Classification of Diseases (ICD-11), which has reclassified it as 'an occupational phenomenon' and defined it as 'a syndrome conceptualized as resulting from chronic workplace stress that has not been successfully managed'.

It's characterised by:

* feelings of energy depletion or exhaustion
* increased mental distance from one's job, or feelings of negativism or cynicism related to one's job
* being less effective in your work.

Let's start out by stating clearly that no one chooses the burnout pathway. If you are suffering from burnout, or feel you are at risk, be assured that it is not a reflection on you as a person. You are not weak, or lacking in resilience or the willpower to succeed, though you may have questioned why you feel so overwhelmed and exhausted when others appear to be managing just fine.

Those who have lived through burnout will tell you it came about because they cared deeply about their work, and wanted to contribute more and to always do their best, but were not supported in their workplace environment, because profits came before people. So the norm was always to do more and go beyond what was reasonable. Alternatively, if you're a solopreneur, startup or small business operator, economic forces drove you to keep pushing harder for longer in order to survive, to remain viable and competitive.

The folly of loving your work too much

If you're thinking the risk of burnout couldn't possibly apply to you because you love your work so much it doesn't feel like work at all, think again. Overwork isn't always something you do out of necessity or because it is expected of you. It can be a choice you make because you're revved up and excited by what you do, forgetting that even the most enthusiastic and dedicated person still needs time out for rest and recreation.

If you're busy justifying to your partner why you need to work every weekend or have pulled out of yet another social invitation because of work commitments, chances are you're a workaholic and, just like an alcoholic, blind to the harmful impact of your behaviour on yourself and those closest to you.

Could you be using your workaholism as a means of escape or, as Josef Pieper suggests in his 1948 classic *Leisure: The Basis of Culture*, to justify your existence?

Workaholics feel compelled to keep on working, but it can be an unhealthy obsession. The good news for recovering workaholics like me is that the Workaholics Anonymous World Service Organisation runs a 12-step recovery program based on the approach used by Alcoholics Anonymous.

Remember, overwork and workaholism are both associated with higher risk of heart disease, stroke and suicide. It's one thing to love your work, but it's never worth dying for. As author Jeffrey Pfeffer puts it in *Dying for a Paycheck: How Modern Management Harms Employee Health and Company Performance — and What We Can Do About It*, 'there can be no trade-off between employee wellbeing and profitability'.

Thriving Mind introduces the strategies revealed by science that can make work and life work better.

 It's time to replace overwork with a better way to be happy, healthy and productive.

Burnout and the brain

From a cognitive perspective, burnout, as its name suggests, has a stark impact on the brain's architecture, a bit like walking through the blackened landscape following a bushfire.

Chronic stress puts your brain under a level of strain it's not designed to cope with. Our stress response evolved to help us deal with immediate, short-lived stressors. When a sabre-tooth tiger parked outside your cave, your brain initiated the fight, flight or freeze response to keep you safe. Once said threat had passed or been dealt with, the stress response could be switched off, allowing you to attend to more pressing needs, like finding your own lunch. Tiger meat sandwich anyone?

The threats we face today are commonly more complex and longer lasting. Having a pack of wolves camped outside your cave for weeks on end meant you couldn't afford to switch off the stress response. Fundamentally, though, the stress response we employ today is much the same as that triggered by our ancestors.

This shows up as your having to remain vigilant to what might be coming around the corner at any moment while still handling last week's oversized courier delivery of change that has yet to be fully unpacked and understood. There's no time to relax or check in to ensure that your new habits, behaviours and thinking patterns are the ones best suited to your needs.

Inside your head the part of your brain called the limbic system, which is involved in the stress response and emotional regulation, goes into hyperdrive. Levels of stress hormones remain high, resulting in a neuroplastic effect causing the amygdalae to grow in volume while simultaneously weakening the links between the amygdalae and those brain areas used for higher executive function and thought. These parts of the brain (called the anterior cingulate gyrus and the medial prefrontal cortex) help keep you sane and on the emotional regulatory safe track.

Remaining hyperalert to continuous threat means you become more reactive and emotionally labile. How many workplaces do you know of where the threat of yet more organisational change is wearing people out and putting them in a more negative frame of mind?

At the tipping point, the red mist descends. Inappropriate, ill-judged things are said and actions taken until all rational good sense and logical, analytical thought are lost. This is dangerous territory. As emotional intensity increases with your stress, it gets harder to stay focused, solve problems or retain information in your working memory. Worse still, you've lost your creative spark.

Sleep becomes elusive and fragmented. Anxieties accumulate and sometimes you feel very low. As you slip further into the downward negativity spiral it gets harder to see any way out of the deep dark hole you have dug for yourself.

It's now only a question of time before all your remaining resources are exhausted. The danger is that even if you've noticed the change in yourself, you park those insights to one side, because you've got work to do.

Ignoring the danger signals nudges you perilously close to the chasm of exhaustion and burnout, increasing the risk of your seeking solace in temporary, artificial consolations such as alcohol, drugs, high-fat, high-sugar foods, and online shopping. *Do you know how close you are to the edge?*

You can identify your risk of burnout using the Maslach Burnout Inventory, first developed in 1981 and still considered the gold standard test, although newer tools such as the Burnout Assessment Tool (BAT), developed by Schaufelli, De Witte and Desart, can also be very useful.

A sense of disconnection and loneliness

To belong is to feel loved, connected to and cared for. It creates a place of safety where we can flourish and be truly happy.

Social connection is vital for wellbeing

Having a strong social support network, with close friends and family, has a profound influence on your health and happiness. It's a major factor in protecting you in the tough times, whether you're struggling through a particularly hard day during which everything goes pear-shaped, or dealing with chronic fatigue, stress and overwhelm. Where's that one Powerball when you need it?

The Powerball might not show up, but your friends will. An enduring sense of disconnection is a problem because it impacts everything, including our health, wellbeing and happiness. Having friends matters because they support us as we deal with the frustrations, disappointments and fear when things go wrong.

It's immensely reassuring to know you've got someone you can call and talk through your challenges and pain with. But what happens when you lack that social support? If you're struggling to deal with the chronic stress of overwhelm, overwork and constant fatigue, chances are everyone else around you is too. You could speak to your manager or boss, but they're always so busy. Their door is supposedly 'always open', yet it's been firmly shut every time you've passed it.

Your colleagues are probably nice people, but you've never had the time to get to know them. No time is allocated for you to get together over lunch. Everyone works in their own little bubble of busy that prohibits opportunities to speak up, to ask for help or to seek clarification. Not wishing to appear dumb, it's tempting to lie low and just pretend everything is okay so when you're next asked, 'How's it going?' you're ready with your practised response: 'Fine thanks', with a twitch of a smile, hoping they won't pry any further.

Whether working in a team, a large department or solo, we all have to fathom how to get along well with others, to try to make sense of why they think and behave differently from us, and to work out a strategy when having to interact with those we find difficult or different.

The reason we form friendships, tribes or groups or live as a family is because above all else we seek connection. Being ignored, rejected or excluded in any way makes us feel really bad. Despite our new technologies, which facilitate superfast connection virtually anywhere in the world, the modern workplace poses ever greater challenges to healthy human connection. Flexible work options, such as working different shifts or working from home or remotely, interstate or overseas in the company's other offices, can mean missing out on training opportunities, social events and face-to-face conversations with your colleagues or management.

When you feel a bit lost, discounted or forgotten about, it hurts. Being deliberately excluded or ignored hurts too. No one likes the thought of being bullied, but the pain of exclusion, as shown in a study by the University of British Columbia, is worse because it creates a feeling of helplessness, leading to greater job dissatisfaction, a higher probability of quitting your job and health problems.

Perhaps, like me, you were brought up to believe that if you've got nothing nice to say about a person, it's better not to say anything. Wrong. It's actually better to say something (just tone down the language) because being on the receiving end of the silent treatment leads us to think we're not worthy of *any* attention and can cause much deeper pain.

The source of support

Your social support network is drawn from a variety of sources, including family, friends and colleagues. Spending around one-third of our day at work, we may spend more time with our colleagues than with our partner and family. This is where workaholism and overwork can wreak havoc on relationships, because our partner at home can be the one feeling left out. So love your job, but never at the cost of losing your family.

Friends at work

Friendships matter in both life and work. One of the major reasons we stay in our job (or not) are the people we work with or for. A Virgin Pulse survey reported that 55 per cent of the 1000 respondents found a positive working relationship with their employer helped them to manage their stress and 60 per cent said this increased their productivity and focus.

A Gallup survey indicated that those with a work BFF (best friend forever) enjoyed seven times the level of engagement at work as those without. Turning up each day to this place called work feels a lot nicer when you know you're surrounded by people you like and who like you back. Is this true for you?

Enjoying strong interpersonal relationships and increasing relational happiness promotes collaboration, contribution and a more positive outlook towards your work and what it provides you. As Sonja Lyubomirsky, author of *The How of Happiness: A New Approach to Getting the Life You Want,* says, 'The centrality of social connections to our health and well-being cannot be overstressed'.

If you're not comfortable with your co-workers, feeling unsupported and generally miserable at work, it's time to address the causes and build a deeper level of connection. By failing to do so you risk an increasing sense of social isolation and loneliness.

With loneliness now recognised as having reached epidemic levels and mental health issues on the rise, it's never been more important to understand how your social brain operates and how to nurture strong interpersonal relationships.

What's making us feel more disconnected?

It all hinges on your perception of belonging and inclusion. You can feel a sense of disconnection despite having thousands of online 'friends' or being strongly connected to a couple of close friends.

Following are some of the contributing factors:

- **Choosing to live alone.** It's important to stress that this is not an issue *unless* you feel you are missing out on social interaction. Being alone is very different from feeling lonely. You may relish the peace and quiet of your own company, especially if it's a rare occurrence or you're an introvert like me who needs your own space to refresh and restore your energy levels. Whether an extrovert, introvert or ambivert, we all like some time alone and other time with our friends.

- **Working off site.** While it sometimes feels great to be able to get some good work done at home without all the interruptions and distractions that are a common feature of most workplaces, working remotely or being posted overseas to a global company office can feel isolating due to reduced opportunities for social interaction, camaraderie and good connection. It's one thing to choose to work off site, and for many solopreneurs and home businesses this is the norm. But being required by changing circumstances to switch suddenly from going to an office to working from home can be a challenge, especially if you have no clearly demarcated work space and you're managing the distractions of children and partner and the loss of connection with the rest of your team.

◦ **The tyranny of distance.** Some projects or work commitments may require you to commute long distances, which can consume several hours of your working day. In some cases it may mean a weekly commute, flying or driving to work on a Monday and hoping to be home by the weekend.

◦ **Spending too much time engaged with a screen.** Today the time spent engaged with a screen takes up an average of 10 or 11 hours a day for some, and this significantly reduces the time available for face-to-face conversation. Zoom and Skype can help boost connection by providing a face to speak to at least, but if your work requires countless hours working with data and spreadsheets, you'll have precious little time to interact with others.

◦ **Spending too much time engaged with your social media.** It's all too easy to lose time updating and interacting on our social media channels. It's been shown that a tendency to compare your own lived experience with your friends' brilliant, exultant posts can leave you wondering why your life isn't like that and trigger greater levels of disconnection and depression.

- **Sleep deprivation**. Have you noticed how being sleep deprived makes you less social? If you're struggling with daytime fatigue, it's hard to find the motivation and energy to do your work well, let alone connect with your colleagues or your family when you get home. And you probably can't face going to your mate's party, even though you value their friendship.

- **Loss of community**. It's not that you don't like your neighbours. You just never get to see them. Working super-long hours means you may go for days or weeks without catching sight of the people next door, especially if they work long hours too. Not knowing your neighbours reduces the sense of community. You'd like to be more proactive, but you don't have the time and you don't know what's on the community calendar.

Disconnection leads to social isolation and loneliness

The most serious consequence of feeling disconnected from other people is the associated sense of social isolation and loneliness that impacts health and happiness. The patients I worried the most about as a GP were those who had little or no social support. Like Margaret, who came to see me every week with a litany of ailments no doctor could keep ahead of. The real reason for her frequent attendance, other than to remind me of my failure to cure the previous week's problem, was she was lonely.

Many GPs and health practitioners I have spoken to have many Margarets on their lists. 'During my years caring for patients,' recalled former US surgeon General Vivek Murthy in a *Harvard Business Review* article in 2017, 'the most common pathology I saw was not heart disease or diabetes. It was loneliness'.

Loneliness leads to feelings of social isolation, a sense that our relationships (where they exist at all) are not meaningful and we are not understood by others. It's a state of emotional suffering that can affect anyone, from the CEO, business leader or busy professional to the student or homeless person, and this social isolation and loneliness are now recognised as a significant public health issue and a growing problem everywhere.

Lonely around the world

It's estimated that loneliness affects one in four Australian adults, with 50 per cent feeling lonely at least one day a week and more than 25 per cent suffering on three or more days. In the US 47 per cent of adults report feeling lonely, a rate that has doubled over the past few decades. The UK government appointed its first Minister for Loneliness in 2018 following the work on the problem begun by the Jo Cox Commission, which revealed that 14 per cent of the British population (9 million people) always feel lonely.

Social disconnection is bad for your health

Here are some reasons why:

1. Research from Brigham Young University found that social disconnection and loneliness are as bad for our health as smoking 15 cigarettes a day, shortening our life span by 15 years.

2. By weakening our immune system, loneliness increases the risk of our catching the local 'lurgy' doing the rounds in the office.

3. The social isolation that means we don't fit in or feel part of the in-crowd leads to a loss of relatedness and being included in decision making or conversations. This is very real and painful.

4. Loneliness can increase the severity of symptoms of depression and anxiety, and make anger management more of a challenge.

If loneliness or a lack of social connection is affecting your health and happiness, there are many ideas discussed in this book that will help you to forge stronger social connections, restore your wellbeing and boost your mood.

Moving towards the light

If you're fed up with feeling unhappy, depressed, lonely or overworked, it's time to bring some positive change to your life. This is absolutely possible and, best of all, you're in control of how you achieve it.

Choosing to thrive is always a work in progress, as we continue to evolve and adapt to our changing world. Luckily this is something you're already good at. The challenge is to move from 'knowing' what needs to happen to making it your reality.

Maya Angelou once said, 'My mission in life is not merely to survive, but to thrive; and to do so with some passion, some compassion, some humour and some style'. Are you ready to be happier, to fully thrive and feel truly connected? Let's take a look at how this can work.

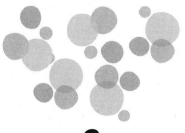

2

Reconnecting to what matters

What is the body? Endurance.
What is love? Gratitude.
What is hidden in our chests? Laughter.
What else? Compassion.
Rumi

Moving towards the light begins with understanding the nature and cause of the current problems you face and how they impact your thoughts, feelings and behaviours. The solution lies in recognising what's been getting in your way and knowing what to do about it while understanding there's no one-size-fits-all answer.

Taking your temperature is a quick and easy way to check if you are running a fever. Now is a good time to check how well you are faring psychologically. In chapter 1 we identified the three key contributors to feeling overwhelmed and out of control as:

- lack of mental wellbeing
- overwork, stress and burnout
- a sense of disconnection and loneliness.

Where did you feel you sat in relation to these challenges? Did any touch a nerve or have you nodding furiously in recognition? Have you forgotten what it's like to feel happy and energised? Are you too tired or too busy for quality time with friends and family? Do you feel you could be in the brown-out zone, on the cusp of burnout? Or have you already got there without having realised it until now?

Acknowledging where you are right now is an important first step. You can take off that superhero cape, because it's not helping.

Shrugging off that cape means reconnecting with what matters, making time and space for the things in your life that help you feel complete. This is not an indulgence — it's essential. You know innately what makes you feel good, strong and grounded. It could be time spent in nature, relaxing with loved ones, going for a swim or taking a long walk. But our culture of working harder and faster, of relentlessly doing more with less, has ground us down, reducing our opportunities for these simple pleasures, relegating them to a short annual holiday (if you're lucky) in which to recover from the overload. It's time to reclaim them.

Your happiness, health and human connection are equally important and interconnected, each supporting the others. They are the holy trinity of wellbeing, the key to your being the best version of yourself: a happy thriving human.

In this book we examine the science behind these three essential ingredients and look at how you can bring more of them into your life.

Happy

When you're in a positive space, you're not only happier but more motivated, energised and eager to take on new challenges. Adapting to change and being more resilient become second nature. You handle life's disappointments and messy upsets more easily and with less residual impact.

Essential ingredients for happiness include:

+ having purpose and meaning
+ practising gratitude and generosity
+ helping others
+ being mindful
+ laughing and playing
+ understanding others' mindsets.

Thriving

Thriving is about enjoying positive wellbeing, feeling energised and seeking opportunities to continue to grow both personally and professionally. You're more open to new ideas, more creative and engaged with all that our multifaceted world has to offer. You're healthy, less prone to sickness and able to shake the common lurgies more readily. Age doesn't slow you down, because your mental and physical capabilities remain strong.

Thriving means making lifestyle choices that support self-care and those little extras that make all the difference to how you interact with the world, such as through music, dance, nature and play.

Essential lifestyle choices for thriving include:

+ rest and recovery
+ sufficient sleep

- healthy eating
- regular exercise
- performing or enjoying music and dance
- time in nature.

Human

Being human is about the quality of your relationships, tapping into your unique qualities of compassion, kindness and empathy in order to encourage greater tolerance, understanding and inclusion. This is about being a good global citizen caring for others as well as our fragile planet.

Essential ways to connect include showing:

- trust and respect
- kindness
- empathy.

Your starting point

Some of these essential elements may already be abundantly present in your life; some may be conspicuously absent. You may, for example, never miss a yoga session or hockey game, but how well are you coping with your lack of sleep? Perhaps you have a healthy diet but can't bear the thought of exercise. You may be convinced you would feel so much better if you got to eat your lunch under the shade of that beautiful tree in the park, but you don't give yourself permission to do this.

If you're ready and open to explore what could be improved, I suggest you rate yourself on each element. If healthy eating is important to you but you know you could do better, ask yourself how you would score on a scale of 0 to 10, where 10 is the best? If you'd currently rate yourself at 7, what can you draw from the book that would take you to 9? As with any renovation project, your remodelling and refurbishment plan, while eminently achievable, is going to require a framework, practice and patience. Knowing where you are starting from gives you a reference point to build on.

Shifting your thinking will be easy or hard depending on how important each topic is to you, your level of interest and your appetite for change. If you're pretty comfy in your armchair of usual, you may be content to enjoy the read and park the ideas until you're ready or you sense the need for change.

If you have the intent but current circumstance, poor timing, fear or uncertainty is holding you back, this book will still provide you with an understanding of things to consider, what's possible and the strategies to put in place when you're ready.

Now you're in the driver's seat, it's time to switch on the ignition and get started.

Part II

Happiness

What it means to be living 'happily ever after'

Whether you're stumbling on, nudging towards or in pursuit of your happiness advantage or following your happiness plan, it appears most of us are seeking something highly prized and elusive.

What makes us happy?

Do we even know what we mean by happiness? Ask around and it's like asking six doctors for a diagnosis — you'll get as many different answers.

Shawn Achor, author of *The Happiness Advantage*, defines happiness as 'the joy we feel when striving for our potential'. Happiness, he reminds us, is what leads us to success rather than the other way around. Too often we are caught up with the idea that we'll be happy when ... [*fill in the blank*]:

⁂ I've saved a million dollars

⁂ I've paid off my mortgage

⁂ I've found my life partner.

Sure, these things will contribute to your happiness, but they're more likely to come about once you've found your happiness.

 Creating happiness is what leads to success.

Martin Seligman, often described as the founding father of Positive Psychology, associates happiness with experiencing frequent positive emotions such as joy, excitement and contentment.

What makes *you* happiest? As in. Truly. Madly. Deeply. Is it:

⁂ enjoying that first morning cup of coffee made by your favourite barista who knows exactly how you like it?

⁂ seeing your child's face light up in delight at some new discovery?

+ spending time with the person you love most in a place of special meaning?

+ that quiet sense of contentment with your lot in life?

+ having a great day at work?

Happiness can be found in the moment or in a more profound, longer-lasting feeling of calm and contentment.

Psychologist Sonja Lyubomirsky proposes that our happiness is 50 per cent predetermined by our genes and 10 per cent by our circumstances, leaving a very helpful 40 per cent that we can influence through our choices and actions. Which is great news!

Happiness, health and relationships

A Harvard study into adult development, launched in 1938, followed the health, lives and outcomes of 724 male teenagers. The group included 268 Harvard sophomores along with 456 disadvantaged youths from Boston's poorest neighbourhoods. About 60 of the original cohort, now all aged in their nineties, survive and still take part in the biannual survey. And 1300 children and spouses of the men have also been included in the study group.

What the study has found is that the single most crucial factor in determining happiness, regardless of age, background or wealth, is the strength and quality of our relationships.

It's no secret: good relationships keep us healthier and happier. Healthy relationships are the lifeblood of our mental wellbeing, reducing the impact and intensity of any physical or emotional pain. The current director of the study, Robert Waldinger, suggests that,

how happy we are in our relationships has a powerful influence on our health ... the best predictor at age 50 of your physical health at age 80 isn't your cholesterol level, but how satisfied you are in your relationships with family, friends and community.

Research into those living in the 'Blue Zones', a term coined by Dan Buettner to describe places where residents are happier, healthier and frequently live well beyond 100 years of age, backs this up. Whether from Icaria in Greece, Ogliastra in Sardinia, Okinawa in Japan, the Nicoya Peninsula of Costa Rica or Loma Linda in southern California, Blue Zone inhabitants embrace strong relationships and family values. As Dan says, 'friends can exert a measurable and ongoing influence on your health behaviours in a way that a diet never can'.

When you're with a close friend or family member, that relationship is strengthened by an increase in the amount of the bonding molecule oxytocin released by your brain. Paul Zak, of Claremont Graduate University in California, has been examining the tricky chicken and egg question: 'Does having more oxytocin make us happy, or do happy people release more oxytocin?' While that debate continues, the research has shown that people who experience bigger increases in oxytocin when receiving a gift are more likely to report greater life satisfaction, to show greater resilience to stressful events, to have a lower risk of depression, to have more and stronger attachments to other people, to be happier and to trust others more.

Oxytocin has also been shown to enhance the pleasure we feel in our social interactions by stimulating the production of the 'bliss molecule' indapamide (also found in chocolate), which has a role in activating the cannabinoid receptors in the brain which heighten motivation and happiness.

Perhaps there's a place for eating more chocolate in the company of friends.

- Where were you when at your happiest?
- Who were you with, and what were you doing?
- How important to your happiness is spending quality time with those who mean the most to you?

Happiness builds resilience

The search for greater happiness is sometimes dismissed as trivial, but it's vital to our resilience to buffer us against our daily difficulties and stress and to reduce our risk of burnout or mental illness.

It works as a positive feedback loop. Building resilience helps create greater happiness, and creating happiness helps maintain our resilience.

Using happiness to build resilience in this way helps to safeguard us from mental distress by reducing our stress levels. When we're happier, we're less likely to take things the wrong way, to be offended by a careless remark or to dwell on what's gone wrong. It's easier to keep things in perspective and reduce symptoms of anxiety or depression.

Being happy and in a positive frame of mind gives your immune system a boost and lowers the level of inflammation in the body, reducing your risk of getting sick or developing heart disease.

The benefits of happiness include:

- better physical and mental health and a stronger immune system
- stronger positive relationships
- a more positive affect (mood) associated with increased optimism, creativity, sense of wonder and curiosity
- less stress and greater resilience
- increased productivity and engagement at work.

And it makes us more attractive to other people because we're seen as being warm, empathetic and caring. Bonus!

Happiness is only one item in your wardrobe of emotions

One of the biggest obstacles to achieving greater happiness is our constant pursuit of it because we think we have to be happy all the time. This is entirely wrong. Feeling happy is a temporary state that can be truly appreciated only when you have experienced the full spectrum of emotions. You feel happy when the person of your dreams has asked you to marry them, or you've landed the perfect job or just because it's a beautiful sunny day. But if your best friend has just confided in you that they've been diagnosed with a terminal illness, or you flunked the uni entrance exam or you overheard someone making unkind comments about you, you will more likely be feeling sadness and disappointment.

Making the most appropriate response by expressing the emotion that best fits a given circumstance helps us to deal effectively with the situation. This psychological flexibility is your emotional intelligence in action. Living a happy life is about responding appropriately to any given circumstance, and knowing when and how to show empathy, concern and compassion.

While trauma is frequently seen as a catalyst for change, experiencing adversity or tragedy isn't a prerequisite to knowing true happiness. Accepting that life is messy and complicated helps you to enjoy the positives and deal more effectively with the negatives. Seeking to avoid pain by denying your reality is a recipe for disaster. Drowning your sorrows, doing drugs or partying all night long to make yourself feel happier doesn't work.

If you've experienced depression, extreme stress or anxiety, and happiness seems out of reach, remember that being unhappy today has no bearing on your future happiness, any more than feeling happy today will prevent you from slipping back into unhappiness in the future.

Creating greater happiness in life and work

Many of us spend more time with our work family than our own family and friends, so knowing how to create greater happiness at work matters. Being unhappy at work because of overwork, toxic working relationships or lack of purpose is a health hazard that spills over into our state of mind in other areas of our life.

Which is why I became a Global Partner in Woohoo inc., a company founded by Alex Kjerulf in 2003 to help spread the message that happiness at work is vital for health, wellbeing and good business. This is no secret. A University of Warwick study, for example, confirmed that the happiest people at work are up to 12 per cent more productive, are likely to stay in their role longer, and take less time off for sick or stress leave.

As Alex Kjerulf explains, 'The main drivers of unhappiness at work are poor leadership, constant busyness and overwork, and jobs with no meaning or purpose'. Is this familiar to you?

Making happiness work better for us

We need to focus on what we KNOW makes us happier, because otherwise we can end up chasing what has the opposite effect. We can easily drift into the negative, the what-ifs and if-onlys.

Stewing over what someone said to us ('They were so *rude!*') or did to us ('Did you see how he cut right in front of me?') keeps us in a negative loop, at risk of catastrophising, magnifying and infecting others in our misery party.

Creating more happiness starts with:

* letting go of the small stuff. Easy to say, harder to do, though it does get easier as we age and start to recognise what's truly important to us and to let go of past failures. Hurrah, an advantage to getting older! There had to be one.

- doing those things that make us happy, tapping into what gave us joy as a kid and giving ourselves permission to play

- focusing on our positive relationships — with friends, family and our social network — to combat the sting of loneliness and cut loose from those relationships that are toxic and harmful.

Are you investing enough time and attention to your relationships, or is busyness getting in the way?

In the next chapters, using the following recipe, we'll unpack what contributes most to being happier and how to recognise what will work best for you.

The best, super-moist happiness cake

Ingredients:

2 cups of purpose and meaning

1 heaped tablespoon of gratitude

6 teaspoons of generosity and helping others

a cloudburst of mindfulness

a sprinkle of laughter and play

1 sprig of mindset

Once well mixed, your happiness cake can be eaten hot or cold but is best created and consumed regularly.

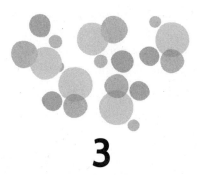

3

Purpose and meaning – for a reason

Happiness is the meaning and purpose of life,
the whole aim and end of human existence.
Aristotle

Why do you do what you do?

We're often told how important it is to know our purpose. But sometimes it's not until we've lost sight of what our purpose is that we come to appreciate what gives us meaning.

After my husband John was headhunted for a new job in Perth, our decision to relocate to Australia felt easy. He was excited by the prospect of working for an organisation he could see was going places, and I was confident I could continue my training as a general practitioner with the ultimate goal of setting up my own practice.

Because the company wanted him to start straight away, John moved first while I completed my contract working in a bustling hospital emergency department in South London. I came out a couple of months later with the idea of taking a three-month break before looking for a job.

But there were a couple of things neither of us had factored into this equation.

With John out at work all day, I had time on my hands for the first time in eight years. With nothing that had to be done other than housework (never my passion), I quickly became bored and homesick. Our funds were limited and other than our two cats I had no one to play with.

After six weeks, frustrated with continually coming home to a weepy and demanding wife, John gently suggested I find myself a job, which I did. It was emergency work again, but that was fine because now I had a reason to get up in the morning. I was reunited with my purpose.

Do you know what your purpose is? What is it that has you bouncing out of bed in the morning? What energises and motivates you to get on with your day?

The brainy benefits of living with purpose

Knowing your purpose enables you to lead a meaningful life.

It boosts longevity

In one experiment, a study that followed up 14 years later on a group of subjects who reported living with purpose found they had a 15 per cent lower risk of death compared with their peers regardless of age or what gave them their sense of purpose. It may be even more important than regular exercise for decreasing your risk of dying early!

The time of discovery is irrelevant. It makes no difference whether you've known since the age of five your calling was to be an astronaut or you didn't discover your life's purpose until you were in your forties. It's connecting with that purpose at some point in your life that matters.

It improves health and wellbeing

Research published in the *Journal of the American Medical Association* showed how, regardless of financial status, gender, race or education level, a strong sense of purpose reduces the risk of developing cardiovascular disease, heart attack and stroke.

Having purpose lowers cortisol levels, strengthens the immune system and elevates wellbeing. How much happier are you when you're living on purpose, experiencing less stress, coping better and enjoying a healthier lifestyle?

Conversely, the sense of being stuck, feeling your life has little meaning, is hugely stressful. Boosting happiness and wellbeing means addressing our physiological *and* psychological needs.

Life purpose is a modifiable risk factor. Choosing to live a life with purpose and meaning ensures better physical and mental health and enhances overall quality of life.

It improves sleep

Between 30 and 45 per cent of older adults report having sleep disturbance of some sort. Research has demonstrated an association between purpose and improved sleep quality, suggesting that tapping into your purpose might prove a useful aid to improving the quality of your sleep.

It boosts cognition

An American study looked at the association between purpose and cognitive function, specifically episodic memory, executive functioning and composite cognitive functioning in adults aged between 32 and 84 years of age. No prizes for guessing their findings showed that those with a sense of purpose scored better on memory and executive and cognitive function at any age.

It changes gene expression

In another study, having a greater purpose in life showed a variable effect on the human genome but was associated with lower inflammatory gene expression and higher levels of antiviral and antibody genes.

It makes us happy

Living a life with purpose and doing things for others are linked to improved health and positive emotion. This emotion differs from the hedonic happiness derived from worldly pleasures such as buying a luxury car or a yacht, which isn't to say we don't enjoy such luxuries, but that they don't produce long-lasting happiness or health benefits.

 Living on purpose keeps you happy, healthy and thinking clearly.

If you're still struggling to work out what you want to do with your life, let's begin by saying there's no need to put yourself under pressure if you haven't yet decided. Your sense of purpose may come later, which is fine because it's something you can build rather than finding it lying around waiting to be discovered.

Seek to identify your passions, values and goals, and write them down. What do you truly care about? Read widely, listen and engage in conversation with others to explore what lights you up. Then commit to living your life fully, with the determination to be your best every day.

Once you know your purpose, it helps you to distinguish between the choices you make because you believe them to be right and worthwhile and those you make because they're easy. Purpose provides you with your moral compass.

Your life's purpose can take a lifetime to create.

Learning to live a more meaningful life full of purpose

Finding meaning in what you do begins with determining what 'one thing' you'd be willing to strive really hard for, accepting sacrifice, stalls and fails along the way. There are a couple of strategies that can help here.

Keep it simple

Less can be more. Fulfilment is easier to achieve once we get rid of all the clutter and stuff that makes us stressed and frustrated.

Focus on what matters

What's truly important to you? Write down the five things that mean most to you. If it's your family, how can you spend more time with them? If it's being of service, look for opportunities to help your community or contribute more through your work. If it's creativity you seek, focus on ways to master your craft, making your hobby a passion.

Your choice of focus changes your brain, rewiring it to help you adopt those thinking patterns and behaviours that will best guide you. Focusing your attention on five things makes it easier not to get side-tracked, or exhausted.

More than a job

You may enjoy your work, but every job has elements we find boring or at least less interesting. You've probably wondered how you can find greater meaning in what you see as mundane or work for work's sake. Data entry is not my thing. Just saying. When I found myself working in a role where that was pretty much the entirety of my work, it was challenging. What made it survivable was knowing that this work was contributing to better health outcomes for Indigenous children, which aligned strongly with my values.

As Dave Ulrich, co-author of *The Why of Work*, describes it, 'Doing meaningful work, whether in a paid or voluntary capacity, provides a sense of living a fulfilling and abundant life. This can be achieved by linking our values, what we stand for, with what is being done'.

This observation is backed up by the research conducted by professional services company KPMG, which drew the following conclusions:

- If your job has special meaning for you — for example, it has a social impact — you'll be twice as satisfied with your work.

- Sharing your story of doing purpose-driven work, recognising and celebrating the meaning and social impact, strengthens pride, engagement and emotional connection to the organisation.

- Leaders who talk about purposeful work raise levels of engagement and morale. If you've ever had the joy of working for a leader who inspires you to do great work because it matters and so do you, what was your happiness rating and sense of fulfilment at that time?

A study by Net Impact found almost half of today's workforce would take a 15 per cent pay cut to work for an organisation with an inspiring purpose. A survey by Calling Brands concluded that purpose was the main driver of recruitment preference and retention, because working for an organisation with purpose saw 65 per cent of employees willingly go the extra mile and remain loyal to their employer.

Delivering your best performance consistently and sustainably is driven by a sense of purpose and commitment to the cause.

See the bigger picture

If your current job isn't aligned with your chosen career path, could it be a stepping-stone towards the work you want?

How can you reframe your perspective to help answer the question 'And what is it you do?' Instead of using your job title to describe who you are, take the macro view.

- Are you a hospital ward cleaner or someone who contributes to the creation of a safe healing environment?

- Are you the manager of a divisional team or a champion seeking to propel others to success?

- Are you a sales recruiter or a dream shaper?

Set yourself some meaningful goals

If reducing waste is your mission, explore different ways to do this in your life and work, and set yourself some achievable targets. If you've got something to say, find a platform from which to share your message, put it out there, get some training in public speaking and commit to the process.

The Japanese tap into something they call *Ikigai*, their 'reason for being', which they believe helps them to live a longer, happier, more balanced life. They determine their big life goal by answering the following four questions:

- **Are you doing what you love?** Seeking work in an area that juices you up, that makes you excited, even though it may be hard, helps you tap into your passion and mission in life.

- **Are you doing something you're good at?** Struggling in an area of work that either is beyond your capacity or doesn't allow you to showcase your skills can be soul-destroying. Reaching mastery in your chosen field, whether as a teacher, a bus driver or an accountant, again taps into your passion.

⚬ **Is this something you can be paid for?** While we all work in order to be paid, the currency here isn't necessarily money. Payment could be in the form of prestige or recognition. This is about identifying your vocation.

⚬ **Is this something the world needs?** If contributing to something bigger than yourself is important to you, then it's an essential factor to consider when determining your work choices. With 94 per cent of millennials seeking to use their skills 'for a cause', there's clearly a growing societal desire to make what we do valuable to others.

Would determining your life goal make it easier to attribute meaning to what you do by making the connection between your goal and what you value?

Create your personal statement of purpose

Try crafting a simple statement around how you choose to live your life each day based on your core strengths, interests and ambitions. Take a moment now to write it down, and review it regularly to check it still holds true. Tweak as needed.

My personal statement is 'To move further each day towards creating a world of greater health, happiness and harmony'.

Be courageous and vulnerable

Leading a meaningful life takes work and the courage to step out of your comfort zone. Being willing to try things out, rejecting the mundane and focusing on the needs of others, can feel hard, even a little scary sometimes. It takes vulnerability too to accept you won't always get things right and to be okay with that.

Finding your purpose and creating a meaningful life provides that deep satisfaction of knowing you are enough, and that you're making a positive difference.

As the late Steve Jobs said, it's about 'creating a ding in the universe'. Are you ready to make your ding?

Your prescription for creating purpose and meaning

- Choose to give, whether it be your time, money or talent.
- Delve deep into your box of interests to discover where your true passions lie.
- Identify what makes you angry, whether it's social injustice, animal cruelty or elder abuse. What and how can you contribute to bringing about change?
- Talk with people, face to face or online, and listen to what they share. What can you learn about yourself and your purpose from the conversations you have?
- Play by your own rules, not those of others.
- Find your joy.
- Appreciate the moment. We have 86 400 seconds available to us every day.

Remember, life is about the journey, not the destination. Finding your purpose and living with meaning makes the ride worthwhile, and makes us happier too.

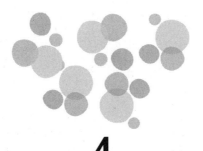

4
Grateful
for gratitude

*Thankfulness is the beginning of gratitude. Gratitude is the
completion of thankfulness.
Thankfulness may consist merely of words. Gratitude is
shown in acts.*
Henri Frederic Amiel

While still only in her early forties, Ruth was doing it tough.
Diagnosed with rheumatoid arthritis as a young adult, she
struggled to deal with the daily fatigue and pain that made it
hard to hold down a full-time job, take care of her children and
feel anything other than tired and sore.

Fed up with swallowing a bucketload of pills each day, she
wanted to find a way to manage her life (and pain) better, which
was when as her GP I suggested she keep a gratitude journal and
try compassion training.

For the first few weeks, the only difference for Ruth was she now
had even more to fit into her busy day, but with encouragement

she persisted. Then around the sixth week she experienced a shift. She still had pain, but it felt more manageable. Her daily activities were still difficult, but she felt less frustrated on those days when her arthritis flared. Her husband reported she was smiling more and was less irritable.

Keeping a gratitude journal and following the practice of compassion gave her back more control of her life and her situation. Expressing gratitude for what she is capable of, despite everything, changed her life for the better.

Being grateful changes your brain: it makes you a happier, more generous person.

Ruth's experience is echoed in research by psychologist Robert Emmons and others, which has shown how gratitude can act as a buffer against the loss of mental wellbeing, general health and vitality that can occur when dealing with chronic medical illness.

Gratitude boosts happiness

In his book *Thanks! How the New Science of Gratitude Can Make You Happier*, Robert Emmons recounts how people who kept a gratitude journal in which they recorded five things they were grateful for once a week for ten weeks enjoyed a 25 per cent increase in long-term self-reported happiness.

Emmons believes the benefits of gratitude to our mental wellbeing include:

- better stress management
- greater self-awareness
- a more positive mood
- more positive emotion and thinking
- improved self-esteem

⚜ reduced toxic emotions resulting from comparing self with others

⚜ increased personal and professional commitment, boosting efficiency and responsibility

⚜ reduced materialistic striving

⚜ motivation to do the right thing

⚜ ability to build stronger social resources (relationships).

Practising an attitude of gratitude makes us happier

In her book *The How of Happiness*, psychologist and happiness expert Sonja Lyubomirsky suggests that when we are grateful we get to savour joy, reducing the burden of negativity in our life and raising both our self-esteem and our effectiveness in handling life's ups and downs.

By making 'counting our blessings' a conscious act, we boost our psychological wellbeing, strengthen social ties and friendships and inspire prosocial reciprocity. Being grateful for what you have today also increases future gratitude, bolstering stress management, building resilience and elevating our overall wellbeing.

 Gratitude is self-seeding.

How gratitude works

Expressing gratitude stimulates the release of dopamine and serotonin, two important feel-good chemicals that enhance mood. Being in a more positive mood strengthens those neural circuits associated with feeling grateful in the right anterior temporal cortex and leads to an increase in the amount of grey matter (more neurons and synaptic connections) in the right inferior temporal gyrus.

Feeling grateful involves our social bonding networks and lowers levels of stress hormones — 'Hey, I feel better now!' — while simultaneously activating limbic activity associated with dispelling negative emotions, so we get better at managing these at a conscious level.

In their study, Emmons and fellow psychologist Michael McCulloch examined the difference between counting your blessings rather than your burdens, comparing three different scenarios over ten weeks:

- The first group were asked to write down things that had annoyed or upset them during the week.

- The second group were asked to express in writing their gratitude for what had gone well.

- The third group expressed no emotional response to their experiences.

After ten weeks, those in the grateful group were found to be more optimistic and felt better about their lives. Interestingly they also made fewer trips to the doctor than the first group.

Other studies suggest more physical benefits of gratitude, including:

- a stronger immune system

- a protective effect on your heart

- a greater capacity to handle pain.

A study from University College London found two weeks of gratitude journalling improved sleep quality and lowered blood pressure. Another study in patients with heart failure found journalling over two months showed reduced markers of inflammation and increased heart rate variability, a sign of improved cardiovascular function.

Being thankful for what you have also helps you sleep better. Reflecting on the positives, alleviating some of your stress and getting a better night's sleep, pays off in greater daytime alertness and a more positive mood. It can also reduce symptoms of anxiety and depression.

What keeps you awake at night? Common causes of sleep disturbance include mental preoccupation, cycling through plans for tomorrow, next week or next year, worrying about past and future events, too many thoughts racing round in your head or feeling anxious — none of which is conducive to achieving the restful state you need for good sleep.

Keeping a gratitude diary requires only three things: a journal in which to jot down your thoughts, a pen and you. The act of writing, rather than using a keyboard or merely thinking, enables your brain to process the information differently. And it's always interesting to look back and reflect on previous journal entries. What were you grateful for on that day and why? Backing up your gratitude with an explanation deepens your perceptions beyond 'I'm grateful for ...'

Cultivating an attitude of gratitude

Saying thank you is never a small deal. It's enormously rewarding to the human brain. It validates what's happened between us, whether a business transaction, an exchange of gifts or a delicious dinner shared with friends. It acknowledges and recognises our actions.

It matters because a lack of gratitude can cost far more than our happiness. When a kind gesture is overlooked, your brain goes into threat mode. Think back to a time when a gift or letter of thanks went unacknowledged. How did this change how you felt about the recipient? Was there a shift in the relationship, a lowering of trust or interest in the other person?

Do the practice

If expressing your gratitude feels awkward, or you're a bit out of practice, take five minutes to practise showing your appreciation. Martin Seligman, author of *Authentic Happiness*, suggests we spend five minutes *every day* writing and sending a letter of gratitude.

Keeping a journal is an easy way to create a habit of gratitude. Take the time to record three to five things you are grateful for in any given 24-hour period, and note why. Committing your thoughts to paper enables your brain to process those thoughts, embedding a neural pattern of gratitude that over time becomes a default pathway and stops you from getting bogged down in less helpful thoughts of negativity, worry and fear.

Positive psychology expert Shawn Achor suggests that journalling for 21 days can lead to six months of greater optimism and that if you're not writing it down, even making a mental note can be helpful.

It's the simple shifts that make a difference. Like choosing to stop replying 'Not bad' when asked by a friend how you are, because the implication is you're not that great either. Changing your response to 'Well, thank you' will shift your mental circuitry towards feeling better about yourself and promote a more positive outlook.

Being more grateful and more vital elevates happiness and success because you enjoy more satisfying relationships, experience less stress and live a more fulfilling and meaningful life.

What a wonderful ROI!

Make it personal

Mandy, a participant in one of my workshops, shared her story of how gratitude had a huge impact on her. She had been with her company for around six months and involved in a big innovation project that had been enormously challenging for everyone involved. When a particularly large hurdle threatened to derail everything, it was Mandy the newbie who stepped up to help resolve it.

She didn't expect to be singled out following the successful outcome. Still, the hand-written card from the CEO expressing their appreciation didn't just make her day; she felt genuinely valued as a member of the team and grateful to be working for such a wonderful organisation.

We typically underestimate the impact of a small gesture of personal thanks on both giver and receiver. It boosts the happiness and wellbeing of both and motivates the recipient to work harder. Which is why stepping away from an offhand 'Thanks guys' and instead delivering a personalised, hand-written note, video or face-to-face conversation is what is remembered and treasured.

If you've ever found yourself buckling under the weight of the hundreds of emails that flood your inbox or despairing under the pressure of meeting yet another unrealistic deadline, you'll know just how easy it is to forget or overlook these small expressions of gratitude. Taking that five minutes, despite everything else happening in your day, matters. As Brother David Steindl-Rast says, 'In daily life, we must see that it is not happiness that makes us grateful, but gratefulness that makes us happy.'

It's time to take back control of our lives, health and happiness, starting with gratitude, because as Robin S. Sharma, author of *The Monk Who Sold His Ferrari*, reminds us, 'Gratitude drives happiness. Happiness boosts productivity. Productivity reveals mastery. Mastery inspires the world'.

Your prescription for the practice of gratitude

- Practise regularly.

- Say thanks more often, and mean it.

- Show your appreciation of others with a hand-written note.

- Do something nice for someone you're grateful to.

- Write a letter of gratitude to someone who has contributed a lot to your life.

- Keep a gratitude journal or a gratitude jar full of notes itemising what you're grateful for and why.

- Start a wall of thanks at work – go public!

- Smile when acknowledging what you're grateful for.

- Host a gratitude party.

- Celebrate your blessings every day.

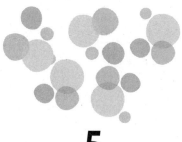

5

Helping out helps everyone

If you want happiness for an hour, take a nap.
If you want happiness for a day, go fishing.
If you want happiness for a year, inherit a fortune.
If you want happiness for a lifetime, help somebody.
Chinese proverb

Having worked hard all her life and reached the age where retirement was expected but not desired, Dennie knew there was something else she wanted to do.

Dennie is one of those people it's easy to be drawn to. She's warm and highly intelligent, has always had the interests of others at heart, and is one of my oldest and dearest friends.

Always a giver, she chose to join an NFP charity close to Redfern in Sydney that provides youth and community services to those in need. For three days a week, she's hard at work matching volunteer tutors with children in need of help to build their literacy and numeracy skills. There is never a shortage of either, but what gives Dennie her greatest joy is seeing 'my kids', as she calls them, rise to the challenge, moving from uncertainty and low self-esteem to greater confidence, feeling encouraged by their progress and rewarded for their achievements.

Dennie has found her volunteering an intensely rewarding experience, and by providing her with a new purpose it has boosted her own happiness.

Do you ever volunteer your time? Hands up! Have you ever signed up to help out for a good cause, and if so, how did it make you feel? Did it change anything in you, shift your perspective or provide greater understanding and insight?

Doing good does us good. Studies have shown that the cumulative effect for someone who's always happy to help is a boost in physical and mental wellbeing, life satisfaction, self-esteem and happiness.

Volunteering is considered an act of free will for the benefit of others. In this arena we're not doing badly by global comparison, with 22.5 per cent of Europeans, 27 per cent of Americans and a full 36 per cent of Australians choosing to 'give something back', whether to help out in a crisis or to support a charity.

Does this make volunteering a lifestyle choice? Take a look at any group of volunteers, and you'll see the smiles, the empathy and the spirit of generosity. Doing something that makes us feel happy is emotionally contagious, creating a warm upward spiral of wanting to help out even more.

Being a 'giver' means focusing outward, coming from a place of service. This translates into a spirit of generosity that has you seeking out opportunities to help. In his book *Give and Take* Adam Grant points out the advantages of being a giver. He believes that givers win the day because by focusing on the greater good and seeking to create success for the group, they convince others to support them, creating a ripple effect of greater generosity. Moreover, the givers who do best give more with greater vulnerability and humility while fulfilling their desire to achieve their own ambitions.

What does giving back look like? It could mean working as a coach or mentor to nurture the ambitions and dreams of others, building a powerful network of support (a big fan base) starting with seeing their potential.

Giving boosts our happy hormones

Generosity as a prosocial act is of great benefit to us because it nurtures trust, loyalty and mutual respect. It also boosts our gratitude and happiness.

In her book *The Giving Way to Happiness*, Jenny Santi reminds us that no matter what our background, the thing that gives us all most joy is the simple act of giving. Helping others boosts our happy hormones. As discussed in the previous chapter, volunteering leads to changes in our levels of oxytocin, serotonin and dopamine. Oxytocin elevates compassion, assisting in establishing trusting relationships. Higher levels of serotonin lift our mood towards the positive, and more dopamine, our chief reward hormone, reinforces the altruistic behaviour that makes us want to turn up again. It's better than consuming your favourite chocolate bar.

The brainy benefits of helping out

Have you ever experienced the 'helper's high'? First described by Allan Luks, the helper's high is that powerful physical feeling or warm glow of increased strength and energy we get from helping others. It comes from the activation of brain centres associated with pleasure, connection and trust that leads to the release of oxytocin and vasopressin.

Helping out involves a network of different brain regions concerned with reward, mentalising (the ability to understand our own mental state and that of others to interpret behaviour) and emotional salience (how our emotions influence what and how we remember), the same areas stimulated by other pleasurable activities such as eating and sex.

Donating to those in need following a natural disaster makes us feel good. Crowdfunding and public pledges of support for events such as Telethon, which raises money for sick kids in Australia, work because they change brain activity in those areas of the brain associated with empathy, social cognition, reward and happiness.

Brain scans have shown even just thinking about giving or donating lights up the brain regions associated with reward. Engaging in generous and altruistic behaviours fosters our sense of wellbeing. As Richard Davidson, professor of psychology and psychiatry at the University of Wisconsin, comments, 'wellbeing is a skill that can be learned' by repeatedly engaging in giving behaviours.

Perhaps you've noticed how being more generous makes you less judgemental, less critical and more tolerant and under-standing of others. In a world of media reports that can come across a tad mean-spirited, self-obsessed or cruel, exhibiting a little more generosity of spirit can go a long way to making the world feel a kinder, happier and safer place to be.

Helping others reduces stress

Stress is something we all have to deal with, but when severe and chronic it can have a detrimental effect on our health. Studies have shown that helping others when we ourselves are stressed helps us to manage our own difficulties and promotes our health and wellbeing.

It's at those times when stress is getting on top of you, and you've ended up in a bad mood or are experiencing poorer mental health that doing something, even the smallest of things, for someone else helps you to cope better.

Yale's Emily Ansell explains: 'Our research shows that when we help others, we can also help ourselves'. She and her team found that while reaching out for social support when feeling low helps us deal with stress, proactively doing something for someone else can be an equally effective strategy. They also discovered that the higher the number of helping behaviours performed, the more significant the boost to mood and mental wellbeing. Helping others buffers the negative effects of stress on wellbeing.

When life and work feel ridiculously busy, leaving you wondering how you are going to get to the end of the day without self-combusting, staying open to support a friend or colleague who needs help can make all the difference. And the virtue of reciprocity encourages them to help you out when it's your turn to ask.

Your empathy validates the other person's feeling and helps them to reframe or reappraise their situation. This practice can increase your emotional regulatory skills, decrease any associated symptoms of depression and improve your overall emotional wellbeing.

Your support doesn't have to involve anything huge or life-changing. Helping out with simple tasks such as running errands, picking up some shopping, driving someone to an appointment, doing some housework or providing childcare makes us feel better and creates a win–win outcome.

What have you done recently for someone else that made a positive difference to you both?

Better health and social impact – win–win

A study from Carnegie Mellon University showed how volunteering for four hours a week for a year could reduce the risk of developing high blood pressure by 40 per cent over four years among older volunteers.

Meanwhile, high school students volunteering in after-school programs lowered their cholesterol, BMI and level of inflammation, indicating that the positive physical effects can occur at any age. Volunteering also increases our empathy and altruistic behaviour and contributes to protecting us from cardiovascular disease.

There can be no doubt that engaging in generous and altruistic behaviours fosters our wellbeing. And there are so many opportunities to contribute through volunteering. Here's just one example.

OzHarvest is a food rescue charity. Founded by Ronni Kahn in 2004, it has grown from a couple of vans to a fleet that collects 'waste' food from supermarkets, hotels, airports, restaurants and other food sources that is then redistributed to those in need.

The scale of the problem being addressed is enormous. An estimated four million Australians experience food insecurity, many of them not knowing where their next meal is coming from, and one million of these are children.

OzHarvest has taken its work a step further by offering training in hospitality to disadvantaged youth to give them a leg up into the job market. At their 'cooking for a cause' sessions young people are invited to assist their qualified chefs to prepare delicious food from the 'waste' food collected. Once a year they run a CEO cook-off where corporates not only dig into their wallets but get into the kitchen to help prepare and serve a meal for 1500 disadvantaged people.

The social impact of the work done predominantly by volunteers is felt on both sides, with appreciation from those in need and a feeling of having contributed in a small way, of having made a difference, by those helping out.

Volunteering can be an adventure, bringing you into contact with people from outside your usual circle, and increasing respect and understanding between people from diverse backgrounds. It's a great way to boost your sense of social connection and provide a sense of purpose.

Helping out alleviates time poverty

One of the biggest obstacles for those considering volunteering is seeing it as yet another 'task' to fit into our already full schedule. Yet our perception of time poverty is largely an illusion. We all have the same 24 hours, 1440 minutes or 86400 seconds available to us each day. It can feel as if we don't have enough time because we're always trying to cram in more. More tasks, more commitments and more time spent checking our social media channels and entertaining ourselves.

With the average person spending over 10 hours a day engaged with a screen, it's little wonder it feels like we never have enough time. Research by James Cook University suggests our tech not only makes our brains work faster, it increases our sense of time passing too quickly. This adds to our stress, which leads to the downward spiral of fatigue, depressed mood and overwhelm.

Choosing to set aside a couple of hours to help out is a golden opportunity to switch off from your phone, computer, laptop or tablet and reclaim your sense of genuine connection.

While valuing and prioritising our time has been shown to make us feel happier, having more free time makes us happiest. Do you have enough?

Your prescription for helping out

- **Spend time or money on someone else.** Giving a five-dollar gift makes us feel happier than spending it on ourselves.

- **Seek out ways to connect with a person in need.** We like to help real people, not statistics, which is why charities will pair donors with individuals to create a stronger connection.

- **Ensure it's your choice to help.** Feeling pressured to donate is a huge turnoff. We want to help of our own volition and see the evidence of how our contribution has made a difference, for example by providing life-saving medical supplies or paying for schoolbooks.

- **Help others to regulate their emotions.** Think of your child throwing a tantrum in the supermarket, or your best friend going through a messy relationship breakdown, or your partner coming home after a horror day at work. Being present, staying calm and showing you care is always a BIG help.

- **Engage in prosocial acts regularly.** Choose to donate something of value to an organisation or association, buy an unbirthday present for a friend or gift morning tea for the office. Creating a circle of helping out is the gift that keeps on giving. As Mahatma Gandhi said, 'The best way to find yourself is to lose yourself in the service of others'.

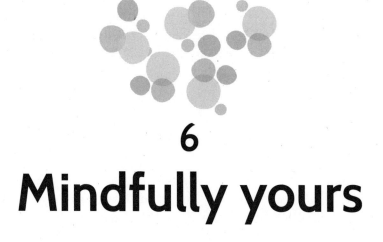

6
Mindfully yours

Look past your thoughts, so you may drink
the pure nectar of This Moment.
Rumi

As a doctor, I've always been good at telling other people what to
do and not so great at heeding my own advice.

Over the years I referred many of my patients with anxiety and
depression for mindfulness meditation classes. It's a technique
that has long been used as a means of reducing stress. My
patients returned sharing how much better they felt, how their
new skill had restored peace, happiness, calm and confidence to
their lives. I was happy for them.

It wasn't until my Gap Year that I decided to give it a try myself
to see if it could alleviate some of the symptoms of anxiety and
depression I was experiencing. Learning to use my breath as an
anchor to stay in the present moment, and to notice my thoughts
without judgement, changed who I am as a person. It made me

kinder and more self-aware. I hadn't realised just how the anger, resentment and judgement I'd been hoarding internally for so long had made me a complete pain in the neck. Great for the physios treating my chronic neck pain, not so great for being a happy human.

Mindfulness has come to mean different things to different people, but the important thing to note is that anyone can learn the skill, and once you have it, like learning to ride a bicycle it remains with you always, even if you haven't used it in a while.

Mindfulness is a mental discipline that with practice teaches you to focus your attention using your breath as an anchor (though it might equally be a guided visualisation, such as focusing on a candle flame). It can be defined as the conscious observation of your thoughts, without judgement, and how these impact your body and behaviour. It deepens your perception of what's going on with other people and in your immediate environment in the present moment. The beauty of it is it helps you regain peace and tranquillity in your own life, while increasing your awareness of others.

Mindfulness is a form of meditation and mental discipline you can practise in the same way you might choose to go to the gym or practise playing your guitar. Research from Yale University revealed how mindfulness meditation decreases activity in the area of the brain called the default mode network (DMN), which is associated with mind-wandering and self-talk, leading to less stress and greater happiness. The DMN is automatically switched on the moment we're not paying attention to a particular task.

At last, a solution to quietening down all that monkey-chatter in our heads for greater peace and calm.

You can be mindful in many ways across a multitude of activities, extending far beyond the time spent in formal mindfulness meditation practice. You are probably already being mindful in all sorts of ways without attributing it to the discipline.

It helps to reduce those moments of mindlessness that can be so annoying and counterproductive. It can be practised formally or informally anytime, anywhere and with anyone, and applied in any situation, whether you're on the bus, preparing a meal or taking time out in the great outdoors. Have you used mindfulness to keep you alert, on track, calm and at peace with yourself?

Today mindfulness is taught in schools, universities, the armed forces, prisons and many businesses, large and small, as a means to better manage stress and emotions, to build resilience and to enhance wellbeing. It has been estimated that you will spend 46.9 per cent of your waking hours thinking about things other than what you are doing right now — either wondering about the future (what's next) or dwelling on the past (what happened). Think how much more useful it could be to increase the amount of time you spend in the present moment — to complete the task you've been working on for the past hour and a half, to be better prepared for what you're going to say in that difficult conversation you've been putting off having, or to notice your partner's worried look.

However you choose to practise your mindfulness, as with any skill, the more practice you put in, the easier it becomes to slip into that meditative space that gives your brain the breathing space required to see yourself and your world more clearly.

Keeping your head when everyone else around you is losing theirs helps your capacity to remain focused and to positively influence the behaviour of those around you. Staying calm and composed in the heat of the moment sounds good, doesn't it? And here's the thing. This is an easy skill to learn because you're already naturally very good at noticing.

There's plenty of science to support the efficacy of mindfulness.

The brainy facts about mindfulness

Many studies have confirmed that regular mindfulness practice, whether through a meditation discipline or through the conscious resolve to be more mindful, supports clearer thinking and better mood. It has also been found to:

- reduce stress, lowering the amount of cortisol and inflammation in your system

- increase the amount of grey and white matter in the brain

- shrink the size of the amygdala, the part of the brain associated with the stress response

- boost your immune system, so you don't get sick as often or as severely

- increase longevity through its effect on cellular ageing

- improve the quality of your sleep

- support improved focus and attention span, which boosts productivity

- improve your ability to learn, memorise and recall

- generate a sense of calm and wellbeing, promoting contentment and joy

- deepen your compassion for yourself and others

- change your perception of pain

- decrease burnout and accidents.

It also makes you happier!

What the monks taught neuroscientists about mindfulness and happiness

It was the Dalai Lama who set neuroscientist Richard Davidson the challenge. Why not use neuroscience to find out more about what contributes to compassion, kindness and wellbeing?

So began a 12-year study in which Davidson invited eight monks who had undergone an average of 34 000 hours of mental training to his lab, where he scanned their brains while they practised compassion meditation alternating with a neutral state.

What he noticed was the high level of gamma brain waves, indicating that the brain was in a highly 'plastic' state, adapting to change and increasing resilience with activation of an area of the brain called the anterior insula, which is concerned with coordinating the brain and body.

Davidson's work showed how mindfulness changes the brain via a neuroplastic effect. This led to the following conclusions:

- Mindfulness meditation is a mental discipline or training that changes brain function.

- The physiological change can be measured.

- Instilling new positive thought patterns intentionally can change your brain for the better.

Our health and wellbeing are highly attuned to multiple different systems of the body, including the immune and endocrine systems.

If you would like to be happier than the average bear but don't fancy becoming a monk, you can influence your wellbeing through mind training, practising focusing your attention to develop a more positive outlook, greater resilience and happiness.

 Mindfulness practice changes your brain.

Strengthen your neural circuits

While mindfulness dials down stress, it increases the amount of grey matter in the prefrontal cortex and the hippocampus, the part of your brain associated with learning and memory, along with the insula and sensory areas involved in hearing and vision. This makes sense because during meditation you quieten down the monkey chatter in your brain while paying greater attention to the sounds around you, staying present and focused on the breath.

It takes only eight weeks of 30-minute daily mindfulness training to show an increase in the density of your cortical grey matter. This is the result of strengthening existing and creating new synaptic connections, making you more effective at dealing with challenging situations and helping you to find greater joy and pleasure.

Meditation reduces brain shrinkage

Our brains shrink naturally with age, but 50-year-old meditators have been found to retain their prefrontal grey matter to match that of 25 year olds. So meditation keeps your brain young.

We spend a fortune on anti-wrinkle creams in an attempt to stay younger looking. Practising meditation keeps our brains more wrinkly (a sign of a healthy brain) and younger looking on the inside.

Stop your mind running away from you

As our workloads and work hours have increased, our ability to handle an ever-expanding cognitive load is increasingly challenged. Perhaps you've noticed the impact on your thinking and emotions during those times when deadlines are looming, you've got too much on your plate and it feels like you're not just stretched but about to snap!

Losing your cool during a meeting with your boss, bursting into tears when your presentation flops, or being so overwhelmed by facts and data that it feels like you're bleeding from the ears isn't conducive to:

+ *positive relationships* — because you're now viewed as volatile and potentially unstable. Can you be trusted?

◈ *high performance* — because your colleagues are unsure if they can rely on you, especially at critical workload moments. Will you let them down?

◈ *smarter thinking* — because you've made a couple of horrible mistakes recently, and the business can't afford any more stuff-ups.

Making good decisions, showing clarity and thoughtfulness in your dealings with your co-workers and clients, while keeping up to date with emerging trends and new technologies, requires a high level of brain fitness. This ensures you retain clear access to your prefrontal cortex, the part of your brain associated with those higher order executive functions including planning, decision making, sound judgement, logic, analysis and reasoning. Achieving this very much depends on your energy level, your focus of attention and your ability to keep your stress at healthy levels so as to help rather than hinder your performance.

If stress is getting the upper hand, you are at risk of overreacting to a comment, interpreting all information through a negative lens or, at worst, developing an associated mood disorder.

I'm not talking about your regular 'Oh my goodness, I just spilt coffee over my shirt' stress, I'm talking about the heavy-duty, soul-destroying, exhausting stress that comes from driving yourself too hard for too long. Your ability to retain access to the prefrontal cortex is now fast receding as your limbic system seeks to gain control.

Your limbic system comprises a number of brain structures involved with your emotions, memory and response to arousal, directing your actions and behaviours. It operates at a subconscious level and is influenced by your values, beliefs and experiences that manifest as gut feelings or intuition. Have you noticed how stress and emotion work hand in hand? The more severe your chronic stress, the stronger any associated negative emotions that now heighten your reactivity to even modest threats.

Eventually something has to give. This is the amygdala hijack, when you're running on pure emotion, which is often when you say or do something you may later regret. At this point your amygdalae (you have one in each hemisphere), the part of the limbic system associated with the generation and interpretation of emotion, essentially shuts down access to your prefrontal cortex (PFC) so you lose access to logic, analysis and reason.

Think of how children behave when they are upset — from toddler tantrums to adolescent door slamming. Their underdeveloped PFC is at the mercy of their amygdalae until their brains reach maturity — around the mid twenties for girls and later for boys. Of course it's not their fault their brains aren't fully mature yet, so we need to cut our kids some slack. Even as grown-ups, learning to tame our brains takes time and practice. Some never fully develop their 'emotional intelligence' — I'm sure you can think of examples!

Don't forget to breathe

In mindfulness meditation we're taught to focus on our breath, bringing our attention back to it whenever we become aware our mind has strayed. While breathing is an automatic process that we don't normally have to think about, we can use our breathing to find calm in a moment.

Think of that tricky situation when everything has gone pear-shaped: you're running late, you've still got a trillion things on your to-do list and now your computer has crashed. What do you do? Do you:

* run around like a headless chook, wailing and beating your chest in frustration?

* press the emergency button to summon urgent, instant assistance?

* take a deep breath? Actually, why not take several?

The simple act of consciously slowing your breathing has a powerful (and instantaneous) effect on the parasympathetic nervous system. It influences what is known as your vagal tone, simultaneously slowing down your heart rate and lowering your blood pressure. The vagus nerve is one of the cranial nerves that links the brain, heart, lungs and gut. When activated it acts like a neural brake, slowing us down. Slowing your breathing causes the level of noradrenaline to fall, helping you to focus better. We use noradrenaline to help us pay attention, but in a highly aroused state it works against us.

A number of breathing techniques are used to restore calm. There are even breath pacing apps to help you create a slow breathing habit. Next time you're feeling highly stressed or anxious, why not try one? The 4–7–8 technique devised by Dr Andrew Weil is based on pranayama or yogic breathing. Start with a slow, deep breath in to the count of four, pause for a count of seven (that's the important bit), then breathe out to the count of eight. Repeat four times.

So simple yet so effective.

Stress-busting with mindfulness

Can it be true? We are fortunate that researchers from Johns Hopkins University chose to do the hard work of sifting through 18 573 meditation studies, locating 47 well-designed random controlled trials that did indeed suggest mindfulness meditation reduces the impact of anxiety and depression. Mindfulness meditation can be a useful adjunct to other treatments.

Meditation as mindfulness-based cognitive therapy has been shown to be almost as effective in preventing relapse into depression as prescribed anti-depressants (44 per cent compared with 47 per cent), while another study showed it alleviated the severity of depressive symptoms by 37 per cent.

Just four days of practice is enough to significantly reduce cortisol, the stress hormone associated with higher levels of inflammation, increased mood swings, higher anxiety and sleep disturbance.

Reducing the threat of stress and mood disorders

Mindfulness practice reduces not only the impact of the symptoms associated with these conditions but also the risk of relapse or developing a mood disorder by helping us to get better at filtering out those unhelpful, unproductive worries that can get stuck on replay in our heads.

Ridding ourselves of those 'what if?' scenarios that disrupt our sleep and wellbeing can help us gain a better perspective of what's really happening, reduce the catastrophising and help us reframe the situation constructively.

Maybe you've noticed how, when stuck in negative self-talk, castigating yourself for making a mistake or being an idiot makes it harder to access more useful thoughts to resolve the problem. This is why our neuroplasticity, which is generally beneficial, can work against us in times of high stress.

If you've always been a worrier or perfectionist or imagined yourself an impostor, tending to err towards stress, mindfulness meditation can help you to:

- successfully navigate those tricky curveballs in life

- enjoy a deeper sense of self-worth

- gain a better understanding of how your mind likes to play tricks on you, tipping you towards moodiness and negativity

- enjoy a better night's sleep, which automatically sets you up to have a better day tomorrow.

Case Study

Vicky, a former patient, was a senior manager who had successfully climbed the corporate ladder. She seemed to have everything in her life and work under control. She was the epitome of success ... except she wasn't.

Having graduated in perfectionism and impostor syndrome with honours, Vicky was struggling in her leadership role. Although the business metrics were looking good and she was receiving accolades for how well her team was performing, Vicky herself was a complete mess.

Putting on that brave smile every morning she felt a complete fraud and was convinced it wouldn't be long before someone tapped her on the shoulder and said, 'You're a fake, get out'. She fretted that mistakes would be made and it would be all her fault. Her outer shell of quiet confidence and professionalism belied the internal struggle she was experiencing with her anxieties, low self-esteem and depression.

She also felt unsupported, because no one knew of her worries, but she was reluctant to speak up because she feared the judgement of others and of being exposed as weak and unworthy of her leadership role. She was deeply unhappy, but the Mona Lisa mask she wore every day meant no one else knew what she was going through.

One day she failed to turn up for work, having been admitted to hospital the previous night with a perforated duodenal ulcer. After the operation she finally opened up to talk about her fears and stress. I suggested she give mindfulness meditation a try.

At first hesitant because she was afraid she wouldn't do it right or it wouldn't work, she eventually agreed to sign up for an eight-week mindfulness-based stress-reduction (MBSR) course based on the work of pioneer Jon Kabat-Zinn, the mastermind

(continued)

Case Study (*cont'd*)

behind the MBSR course designed to assist in the treatment of pain and depression.

Three months on and Vicky felt like a new woman. She was sleeping better, and her anxiety levels were well under control. Now feeling in control of her thoughts, she was once again enjoying her work. She chose to continue with her daily mindfulness meditation practice and started to encourage other members of her team to try it too.

Using mindfulness to reduce your stress helps to counteract the negative and fearful thoughts generated by the limbic system, making them less reactive.

 Mindfulness is the gift that keeps on giving.

Mindfulness can be helpful in every workplace for alleviating symptoms of high stress. It doesn't eliminate unpleasant sensations; rather, it changes your relationship to them. But it isn't a panacea for the underlying causes of workplace stress, including long working hours, excessive workload, lack of autonomy, lack of flexibility in working hours, insufficient down time and rest, bullying, unrealistic expectations, and lack of support and resources. These issues need to be tackled separately.

Mindfully managing the upside of stress

We usually talk of the downside of too much stress, so it's easy to forget just how useful stress is to us. It prepares us to respond to change in our environment. It raises our performance through the release of our catecholamines, the stress hormones that at healthy levels provide us with that little tingle of anticipation or sense of excitement, helping us to step up to the challenge and grow professionally and personally.

As psychologist Kelly McGonigal, author of *The Upside of Stress*, reminds us, 'Stress can transform fear into courage, isolation into connection and suffering into meaning'.

Using mindfulness to lean into stress, accepting it as normal, expected and often surprisingly helpful, increases our wellbeing. lowers the impact of chronic stress on our system, and keeps us healthier and happier.

It takes a reframe to discover why the stress you feel relating to your elderly parents, who need to be moved into aged care soon, is a normal response to finding the best solution in a difficult situation, because you love them. Or to dissipate your anger after a meeting that ended badly, because you care about your integrity and professionalism and doing the right thing by others.

Mindfully paying attention to your thoughts, feelings and emotions helps you to nurture stronger, more positive relationships in life as well as work.

This works by:

- **mindfully coming off autopilot**. Give your complete and undivided attention to the other person. Tune in to your gut to be aware of any way in which you may be reacting defensively or prejudging the other person. Attention is a two-way street, so give yourself permission to pay attention to what is being said and show the other person you're fully listening.

- **increasing awareness of when you're emotionally off course**. This means getting better at recognising the danger signals when you're reacting in an unhelpful way. Mindfully accepting what has happened (whether good or bad) allows a conversation to take place that increases mutual understanding.

- **stimulating greater empathy**. Mindfulness affects the insula, the part of the brain concerned with empathy and compassion, keeping you aligned to finding a resolution despite differences and promoting greater tolerance and understanding.

The how and when of mindfulness meditation

It's easy to overthink and overcomplicate meditation. Adopting the KISS principle (keep it simple, stupid), the best way to learn is to sign up for a course to embed the practice. Learning mindfulness meditation isn't hard. The challenge is making it part of your everyday schedule, something you do because it's part of your wellbeing strategy that's as natural as brushing your teeth every day.

Having made the decision, what equipment do you need?

Just yourself and a quiet place where you can sit or lie down and be comfortable, without fear of interruption.

What, no orange robes or mountaintops?

No, these are not required unless you feel so inclined. The easiest way to start is to sit in a comfortable chair with your back straight (imagine you have an invisible thread holding your head up straight). Keep your feet flat on the floor, and your arms relaxed across your lap. Then either close your eyes or look down with a soft gaze and focus your attention on your breath. Though your breathing is automatic, by bringing your conscious awareness to it, you can use it as a single point of focus.

During training, you'll be encouraged to undertake a home practice of 45 minutes. Don't be surprised if you find yourself falling asleep in those initial sessions. The length of your practice sessions after the course is up to you. Whether you choose to meditate for five minutes or an hour is a personal choice, though you can expect greater benefits from longer sessions.

The when of your practice is also a personal choice. Morning, evening or sometime during the day, whatever best suits your schedule, then make it a consistent habit.

What, every day?

Again, up to you. Every day is great; several times a week is fine. There may be periods when you stop the practice and other times when you spend more time on it. Maybe you can manage 30 minutes on some days and only ten on others, but regularity will serve you best.

What if I fall out of practice?

Don't worry, this is not uncommon. As my meditation teacher Eric Harrison advised, learning mindfulness meditation is just the beginning. The hard part is to make it a regular part of what you do on a daily basis. There will be times when you practise religiously every day and times when you take a break. What counts is knowing you can always draw on the skill when you need to.

How do I know I'm doing it right?

If you've followed the basic principles, you've got it right. Don't expect to be able to empty your head of thoughts — that isn't possible. Some sessions will feel great, some not so much if your chattering monkey mind is being particularly noisy and intrusive. Every time you notice a thought pop into your head, acknowledge it, allow it to float by and bring your attention back to the breath, over and over again.

Counting breaths can sometimes help — try counting up to ten then back down to zero. You might prefer to listen to a guided meditation using an app, or you might opt for silence with a timer.

Can I do this at work?

Absolutely. Some workplaces provide a meditation room; others hold a mindfulness session at the beginning of the day or during the lunch break, or you might create your own space and time.

Getting support from your colleagues by joining a WhatsApp or Facebook or intranet group can help maintain your motivation by allowing you to share your wins or your need for encouragement.

Can I use an app?

There are a large number of meditation apps available. Find one that suits you. Some provide guided meditations; here you'll need to find the right 'voice'. Others provide different sounds. Many include a selection of different time lengths, useful for those days when you can afford only 10 or 15 minutes. Some apps are designed to encourage you to keep coming back by counting how many successive days you have meditated, prompting your self-competitive spirit: *Come on Jenny, don't break the chain!*

Interestingly, some of these meditation apps are now being repurposed as sleep aids. Meditation is known to help improve the quality of sleep by reducing anxiety. If sleep is an issue for you, why not check out a sleep meditation app to see if it will help you?

Wouldn't I be better off just getting more sleep?

Getting enough sleep is certainly a great way to help alleviate symptoms of anxiety and stress, and if you are able to consistently achieve the 7–8 hours of good-quality uninterrupted sleep most of us need for best functioning, then Bravo. But if sleep is an issue for you, and we'll talk a lot more about sleep in a later chapter, learning mindfulness meditation can be a huge help. Here you're using your conscious awareness to develop the skill needed to relax and quieten the mind in preparation for sleep. By making mindfulness meditation a regular practice, you're training your brain to better manage the day's stress. A study that compared the effectiveness of mindfulness meditation to sleep education in subjects over 55 years old showed the former resulted in more improved sleep and less daytime fatigue. Meditation boosts the production of the sleep hormone melatonin and the feel-good hormone serotonin lowers blood pressure and slows the heart rate.

Falling asleep is a fairly common response when first learning mindfulness meditation. In my early days of practice my husband would not infrequently find me lying on our bedroom floor snoring my head off. 'Meditation practice going well?' he would ask with a smile as I came too, realising I hadn't quite achieved the relaxed meditative state I had sought.

The Indian spiritual leader and founder of the Art of Living Foundation, Gurudev Sri Sri Ravi Shankar, describes the difference in this way: 'Wakefulness and sleep are like sunrise and darkness, while dreams are like the twilight in between. Meditation is like the flight to outer space, where there is no sunset, no sunrise — nothing!'

From formal to informal – introducing the mindful moment

Not all mindfulness involves formal meditation practice. You can also take a consciously mindful approach to an everyday task, slowing your mind down and engaging all your senses. We are frequently unconsciously mindful. Think about when you take that moment to pause and savour your morning cup of coffee. Feel the heat of the cup, the shininess of the porcelain and the wonderful aroma. Notice the pattern your barista created just for you on the crema and the taste as the coffee touches your tongue.

Or it might be a moment when you really take notice of something you normally do without conscious thought. Like the way you chop the vegetables for dinner, or brush your hair, or slip off your shoes to stand barefoot on the grass.

Adult colouring-in books that were all the rage a couple of years ago are great for adopting a mindful approach to a task. When visiting a design studio for a meeting with the CEO, I was taken past the lunch area where several employees were deeply engaged with their colouring in. It's perfect for a creative environment where a calm and alert mind can trigger more innovation and insight.

Creating a mindful moment is useful:

- before answering the phone
- before a difficult phone call
- before having a difficult conversation
- before responding to a complaint
- when recognising your rising level of frustration or irritation with your partner, colleague or client is getting close to the danger zone
- before meeting with a new client
- when stuck in a boring meeting
- when stuck in traffic
- while commuting to and from work on public transport
- during your lunchbreak
- while exercising
- when preparing a meal
- while doing the dishes
- while standing in the queue at the supermarket checkout
- before opening the front door after getting home from work.

At any given moment, by taking a step back to notice what's happening for you, what's going on around you, and choosing to stay in the present moment, your practice creates a mindful ripple effect that spreads naturally to other aspects of your life and work.

Whether a moment or a formal practice, mindfulness is a skill that can be used anywhere at any time to help keep you (and others) safe.

Mindfulness is not the solution to all our ills, and it's not for everyone. But if stress, anxiety and overwhelm are wearing you down, and you're willing to give it a try, it might be just the thing to reinstate the calm, happier, confident you.

Your prescription for greater mindfulness

- **Make it a choice.** Your decision to be more mindful is the first step to greater self-awareness.

- **Seek ways to make mindfulness helpful to you.** Is it about alleviating some of your stress, raising your level of happiness or being more attentive to what's happening right now?

- **Create your mindfulness space.** Choose a place that is quiet, calm and relaxing, somewhere you'll want to visit more often.

- **Put in the practice.** As with any new skill or habit, the more practice you put in, the greater and quicker the benefit. It's the consistency of practice that counts.

- **Use it for the greater good.** Being more mindful helps you to regulate your emotions, set judgement to one side and be open to greater tolerance and understanding of what's happening with others.

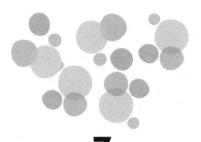

7

Laugh and play makes your day

*A good laugh and a long sleep are the two best cures
for anything.*
Irish proverb

One aspect of our health and happiness that can be overlooked is the benefit of laughter and play.

When I worked as a junior doctor in an emergency department in London, we never knew from one shift to the next, from one moment to the next, what would unfold. As a team, we responded reflexively in the way we had been taught to do, whether treating cuts and broken bones or seeking to save a life. We were always ready to leap into action when the cardiac arrest alarm sounded, as well as to allay the fears and anxieties of our patients and their relatives and to manage our own emotions.

I almost died laughing

We developed what might have been seen as a rather macabre humour, finding the humour in what others would have seen as distinctly unfunny. But it helped to keep us sane by counterbalancing the emotional intensity of dealing with so much trauma and death.

When we laugh a lot, our cortisol levels drop, and we feel more in control of our situation. Laughter helps alleviate the misery of discovering you said something that unintentionally caused offence. It reduces the shock and consternation you feel after realising you sent *that* email to the wrong person. It diminishes the embarrassment of falling flat on your face in front of the person you've been trying so hard to impress. Or after realising you've been walking around with your skirt hitched up into the back of your knickers all afternoon.

Have you ever used laughter as a means of relieving pent-up tension, or defusing a situation you could see was otherwise going to end in tears?

Laughter really is the best medicine

Research in gelatology, the study of laughter, has shown that a rip-snorting belly laugh has myriad health benefits. Let's take a look at some of these.

 ## Laughter boosts your immune system.

Can laughter really keep you well? Studies by Dr Lee Berk and colleagues at the Loma Linda University of Allied Health and Medicine have shown how laughter promotes the increase of antibodies and activates the body's protective cells including our 'natural killer' cells, which are able to check the growth of tumour cells, at least temporarily.

Perhaps you've noticed what a difference a positive outlook and good social support can have on how well people recover from illness or cancer treatments or dealing with loss or bereavement? The connection between mind, body and emotions is very real. The new field of psychoneuroimmunology (PNI) is exploring the interaction of psychological stress and the immune and endocrine systems. One metanalysis of 300 studies shows how acute stress strengthens the immune system but chronic stress weakens it.

Worries about paying the bills, relationships or job security can trigger stress-related disease; laughter, a powerful stress buster, can come to the rescue.

This means having a good belly laugh increases our resistance to disease, but only if we laugh out loud! A silent snigger doesn't produce the same effect. When did you last have a rip-snorter that reduced you to tears and made your ribs hurt from laughing so hard?

It's good for your heart

Dr Michael Miller, director of the University of Maryland's Center for Preventive Cardiology in Baltimore, showed how the associated endorphin release from laughter influences the release of another substance called nitric oxide. Nitric oxide increases blood flow, reduces inflammation, inhibits platelet clumping and reduces the formation of cholesterol plaque.

That's why choosing to watch *Saturday Night Live* rather than the latest horror flick could be a good move towards reducing inflammation and boosting coronary blood flow.

Miller suggests that in addition to our exercise prescription we need to add 15 minutes of daily laughter. This could also be good news if you've been advised to take a statin for your high cholesterol. Maybe a bit more laughter and play is in order. The American Heart Association actually recommends laughter for a healthy heart.

It increases longevity

The good news for women is that a Norwegian study of over 53 500 women found that women with a strong sense of humour despite illness, especially cardiovascular disease and infection, lived longer. A higher score on humour translated into a 48 per cent lower risk of death from all causes, a 73 per cent lower risk of death from cardiovascular disease and an 83 per cent lower risk of death from infection.

For men, the efficacy of humour in cases of infection is evident, although not for cardiovascular disease. Sorry guys, life isn't always fair.

It reduces stress

Watching a funny show has been shown to reduce levels of the stress hormones cortisol and epinephrine. This discovery led Berk and colleagues to develop Laughercise©, using laughter to prompt the body to respond as if you've engaged in moderate physical exercise. It elevates mood, decreases stress, lowers your systolic blood pressure, raises HDL, the good sort of cholesterol, and, as already mentioned, boosts your immune system. What's not to love about a little more Laughercise© in your world?

A hearty laugh can also help reduce muscle tension for up to 45 minutes. Think how much less stressed and tense you'd feel from laughing a little more often during the day.

Sharing a laugh in a situation where anger and hostility are brewing can help each side keep things in perspective and move towards a negotiated settlement, reducing the risk of a stalemate, bitterness or resentment. How important is this when you're in a situation everyone is finding difficult?

If frustration and fatigue are getting you down, laughter can make your day feel a whole lot better.

Using self-effacing humour ('I'm such a clot to have made this mistake!') also shows others you're only human, which can help to break down barriers and strengthen relationships, trust and understanding.

Do you incorporate humour into your life and work for better stress protection?

It reduces symptoms of anxiety

Nervous laughter in the face of fear is something many of us are prone to. That nervous titter or giggle is our brave attempt to overcome the anxiety—say, of being in an awkward social situation. It helps us to regulate our emotional state.

Laughing can help us to express our true feelings as well as alleviate pain. Okay, this is more about using humour and laughter as a distraction and raising pain thresholds by elevating endorphin levels. But if it works, go for it!

When immunising small children, I found it really helpful to use my best smiling, happy face and peek-a-boo technique to help relax both parent and child. Speed of delivery was of the essence, so the child was left wondering what just happened while the syringe and needle were deftly disposed of and the smile and laugh routine maintained. Alas, this never seemed to work quite as well with adolescents and adults, who generally saw through the ruse.

We remember the funny

Do you remember when ...? It's those events and stories, whether simply ridiculous, slightly embarrassing or side-splittingly funny, that we remember far longer than any of those data-heavy, death-by-PowerPoint presentations. Having a laugh or enjoying the humour in a situation stimulates our short-term memory. We're better at learning and retaining the new information because it lowers stress hormones and our blood pressure, boosts our mood, raises endorphins, stimulates dopamine release, strengthens the immune system and shifts brain wave activity towards more gamma waves known to benefit memory and learning.

Researchers from Loma Linda University believe laughing — say, by watching something funny on YouTube — every day is a fabulous way of retaining our learning ability and delayed recall as we age.

If you're losing your car keys too often or having problems remembering items because of the pressure or work-related stress you are experiencing, perhaps there's a place for incorporating more funny cat videos into your work day.

It makes us more creative

The late Robin Williams was one of my all-time favourite comedians. One study showed how watching Williams with some of his great one-liner jokes led to a 20 per cent increase in creative problem solving when working with puzzles.

Have you ever found you've had more great ideas when relaxing and laughing with friends? Does it help you let go of your inhibitions and be more spontaneous?

What role does humour play in your life in stimulating more creative thinking? With innovation teams under constant pressure to come up with new ideas in the knowledge that many of their prototypes will be abject failures, staying in a positive frame of mind using humour can keep your imagination firing while reducing the pain of knowing not all your brilliant ideas will come to fruition.

Boosting happiness with laughter yoga

I confess when I first heard about laughter yoga, the thought of standing around with a group of people faking laughing sounded quite ludicrous. Putting my cynicism aside I chose to follow my curiosity to discover more about this unlikely method for enhancing happiness from Peter Schupp, who has been running classes for the public and corporates in Perth for a number of years.

Laughter yoga was introduced to the world by Dr Madan Kataria. Peter explained how it is an exercise that incorporates clapping, breathing and moving while doing fake laughing until real laughter takes over. He says it boosts resilience by shifting our perspective towards the positive and reducing negative emotion. He sees the benefit of this for the workplace, where stressed-out workers can alleviate some of their stress so they are better placed to handle their many daily work challenges.

A pilot study at Deakin University backed this up. Working with two Melbourne businesses, the study showed how a single session of laughter yoga was an effective intervention to temporarily increase wellbeing, with an associated drop in stress levels, and a reduction in anxiety and depression. And those who started with the lowest level of wellbeing before the class derived the greatest benefit.

What about having a laughter session to increase your level of endorphins and put yourself in a better mood? Maybe this is a good example where to fake it until you make it does pay off.

How can you learn to laugh more?

Here are some simple ways to bring more laughter into your life.

1. Set the intention

As with any new habit, it's about setting the goal, then creating a framework to make it happen. Setting yourself the challenge includes establishing a time frame — say, 21 or 30 days.

What does your goal look like? Is it to challenge yourself to see the funny side of a situation more often? Is it to smile more often each day? Decide what it is, write it down (to glue it into your brain circuitry) and post it where you will be constantly reminded of your goal.

2. Tell others what you're up to

Having support and someone to keep you accountable will help. If they know you're booked to go to a laughter yoga class on

Thursday night, they'll expect you to go — no excuses! Why not get them to come along with you and join in the fun.

3. Reduce your negative influencers

This can include other people — why hang out with those who bring you down? If friends and colleagues are lifetime members of the BMW (Bitch, Moan and Whine) club, it's probably time to branch out to seek new associations that inspire you and make you happy.

Be mindful of your exposure to the news and social media. With so much negativity in the press, it can be hard to find a good news story. One way to manage this is to manage your input. Just because the news channels run 24/7 doesn't mean you have to be tuned in all the time. Counterbalance the gravity of the news by also listening to lots of happy music, positive podcasts and funny shows.

4. Seriously, it's about finding the happy medium

Yes, life and work are serious, but if you're locked into all that serious business without ever lightening up, it's a recipe for getting trapped in a negativity rut. Let's face it, if you can't step back to relax and smile more, you're less attractive to others. Who wants to hang around someone who's always super intense and serious about everything?

5. Get better at laughing at yourself

If you're always giving yourself a hard time for making a mistake or being less than perfect, it's time to change perspective channels and turn that embarrassment or shortcoming into an opportunity for self-compassion and laughter. Hanging out with friends who make you laugh is guaranteed to keep you in a good mood and keep you laughing. As Charlie Chaplin said, 'A day without laughter is a day wasted'.

But laughter on its own is like butter without bread. Being playful is the other side of the laughter coin, and when taken together they bring joy and delight, as well as greater health and happiness.

The power of play

As George Bernard Shaw reminds us, 'We don't stop playing because we grow old, we grow old because we stop playing'. How does being playful make you feel? Light? Content? Expansive? Generous? Interested?

We can learn a lot from children. Their natural spontaneity, curiosity, creative spark and joy in fun helps them to make better sense of their world and makes them more effective learners. It's also contagious.

When we reach adulthood something weird happens: the busyness, overwhelm and exhaustion associated with life and work often cause us to lose that sense of playfulness.

While sleep and lifestyle choices are important, so too is the choice to laugh and play more as a stress-busting strategy that increases resilience against potential burnout. All work and no play doesn't just make Jack and Jill dull people; it can lead to boredom, lack of initiative, loneliness, anxiety, depression and unhappiness, none of which are conducive to doing great work.

The brainy benefits of play

Why should kids have all the fun? Play at any age brings a number of cognitive and health benefits, including:

- increased creativity
- improved critical thinking
- improved brain function, including problem solving
- better memory and increased neuroplasticity
- stronger positive relationships
- increased mental wellbeing

- improved physical health

- lower stress levels

- increased happiness.

Let's look at how play can help us in everyday life.

Play helps to dispel negativity

As those negative thoughts accumulate like storm clouds on the horizon, symptoms of depression can start to sneak up on you. While depression can have a multitude of contributing causes, what keeps us stuck is that ruminative thinking that has us replaying the same negative thoughts over and over while avoiding taking action to overcome them. *I'm such a loser. No wonder I've never been successful at anything. I've wasted so much of my life. I'm ugly and worthless. No wonder my partner cheated on me.* Breaking the pattern of negative self-talk is helped by distraction, one source of which is play.

Come and play!

I know, this might feel like the last thing you want to do. You're so busy. You've got a million and one items on your to-do list. You're tired (and, admit it, a bit grumpy). You're coming up with every excuse under the sun why you can't or won't play. But play can liberate you from those unhelpful thoughts and stifling negativity, freeing you up to adopt a healthier perspective and lighter mood.

Give yourself permission to show up and give play a whirl, whether with a structured game, free play, or a gadget or toy.

Play as a disruptor

Play brings change. It disrupts the usual and takes you to a new place where you've got something else to think about. It loosens the straps on your imagination and creativity and helps you adopt a fresh perspective. Now you can see the different options and possibilities available to you more clearly.

Letting go can feel a bit scary. Whether you're about to dive into a deep pit of plastic balls, zoosh down a water slide or sneak a ride on the swing in the children's playground, this is the time to feel the fear but rise triumphant, having had a go.

Play is fantastic for raising confidence levels — 'I didn't think I'd be able to do that!' — and is a fabulous stress buster. When you're feeling under constant pressure, play provides a powerful stress release valve to let you blow off steam.

If you're not sure about launching out on your own, team play can help you feel safe *and* unleash your competitive side. Those team-building days are designed for you to get to know each other better, using different activities in which you may be pitched against each other in a fun and playful way. The Escape Room, Zooscursion, Great Race, Treasure Hunt and Bike Building competitions are examples of team play I've seen work brilliantly in a number of different workplaces. Has your experience of these helped you feel better understood as a person? If so, how can you apply this knowledge in order to engage with your colleagues more often in a lighter, more playful manner?

Play as a diversion

Play, like laughter, can help you better manage chronic pain or difficult health ailments, helping you to cope better and boosting your mood. When lost in a game or creating your next artistic masterpiece, worries become less insistent and anxiety can take a short break. Play allows your mind to let go of those negative thoughts and enjoy the novelty of doing something different. Make it a fun challenge (great for driving neuroplasticity) without the pressure of it being a chore.

Play forges strong social bonds

Joining a club or signing up to a sports association is an opportunity to meet new people and create connection with people you might not often come across in your daily life and work. Being an all-rounder by making work just part of your life, not the majority stakeholder, is a great way to boost health, happiness and wellbeing. Is it time you reconnected with the feeling of joy and exhilaration that comes from play?

Use play to make work work better

Psychiatrist Stuart Brown, founder of the National Institute for Play and author of *Play: How It Shapes Our Brain, Opens the Imagination and Invigorates the Soul*, reminds us how 'work does not work without play'. Why? Because, as he explains, play helps us to deal with our various challenges, promotes mastery and helps us to be more creative in our outlook, leading to greater joy and satisfaction.

 Play and work are mutually supportive, not polar opposites.

Play improves decision making and creative thinking

Problem solving and decision making can take up a large amount of your regular thinking time. Higher order thinking (HOT), using your executive functions of logic, reasoning and analysis, consumes a great deal of mental energy so finite resource requires careful management across your day. Sometimes you'll find the answer you seek by taking the HOT route, weighing up the pros and cons, carefully considering all the information available, but sometimes not.

Sometimes, rather than pushing on and getting more mentally fatigued and frustrated, it's time to draw on your creative, playful side, letting go of focus to come up with more insight. Board games such as Pandemic, Catan, Citadels, Dominion or Ticket to Ride require you to think differently, and it's the out-of-the-box thoughts that lead to more divergent thinking.

Play makes us more productive

Have you noticed how much more engaged and focused you are when you're in a more playful mood, and how time passes much more quickly? Little wonder it makes us more productive.

As psychologists René Proyer and Willibald Ruch point out, 'playfulness may serve as a lubricant in productive work situations'. Sounds intriguing! Naturally it requires more than one player. Adopting a more playful attitude enables exploration of new ideas, experimentation, trial and error. How could this help you be more adaptive and responsive in how you go about your daily tasks?

Your prescription for more laughter and play

- **Choose to laugh more.** Start with a smile, let out a chuckle and move up from there.

- **Look for the ridiculousness in a situation.** Lighten your pain by choosing to laugh and release all that muscular tension.

- **Spend more time with young children or animals.** Seeing them having fun and participating in their play will quickly help put a smile on your face and soon have you laughing. When did you last play 'let's pretend'?

- **Seek the funny.** Watch funny YouTube clips, comedy sitcoms – whatever tickles your funny bone.

- **Choose a playful approach to explore new ways of thinking and doing.** This is about taking a risk and running with it. Whether it works or not isn't the point.

(continued)

- **Choose a playful lens to lighten your perspective.** Worry less about 'what would people think?' and get on with the task at hand. Playing safe is about maintaining your self-confidence and self-esteem in everything you do.

- **Create your play box at home.** Include all those things you love to play with, whether it's board games, pens, paints, paper – whatever you find fun.

- **Turn your work into a game.** This intellectual playfulness frees you up to get more creative and make your work more interesting and stimulating. Why not share some memes with your colleagues and invite them to play along? It doesn't have to take a lot of time or be disruptive to your work. Think of it as a playful interlude or recess!

- **Schedule some play dates in your calendar.** Give yourself permission to have a 'play day', and spend the time as you wish – painting, writing, cycling around the park or whatever you want.

- **Change a stressful event into an opportunity to respond in a playful manner.** If someone's got you barking mad, you could jump up and down or try to see the funny side of the situation.

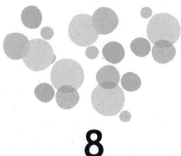

8
Mindset – dial up the positive

Your beliefs become your thoughts,
Your thoughts become your words,
Your words become your actions,
Your actions become your habits,
Your habits become your values,
Your values become your destiny.
Mahatma Gandhi

It was my psychologist who jolted me out of victimhood. Recovering from burnout, with the associated mental distress and trauma of losing my practice, meant having to deal with a range of emotions that I'd spent a lifetime trying to suppress. I was dealing with a hollow kind of numbness and disbelief compounded by feelings of shame and anger.

I needed help, but I wasn't happy about needing it. I was desperate for support but uncomfortable and feeling selfish about reaching out.

I wanted to blame someone, and my former business partner was in the direct line of fire. I was a victim and playing the role well enough to earn an Oscar, or at least a Golden Globe nomination.

Bit by bit, week by week, as our uncomfortable conversations continued, my psychologist teased out ways to get me to tell my story from a survivor's perspective. This was new territory for me. I was still grieving my loss, trying to make sense of what had happened and looking for a way to get back to normal, whatever that was.

It was his question 'And how did you contribute to this story?' that provided the jolt I needed. My first thoughts were *How dare you! I'm the victim here, don't you see? Aren't you supposed to be on my side, helping me here?* Yet after a moment of quiet reflection the insight struck me that it had indeed been my dogged commitment to putting work above everything else, including my own needs as a mother and a wife, that had played the greatest part in my downfall. Ouch.

My Anglo-Saxon work ethic demanded that I work harder than anyone else and always go that extra mile. This meant I was a time bomb of my own making. It was time to let go and to heal.

Victim, survivor, thriver

As victims we are stuck. We are suffering, and though it hurts, we hold our pain close to our chest, unwilling or unable to let it go. We're mortally afraid of what's happening, of what our future might hold, and we continue to listen to replays of our negative self-talk and limiting self-belief.

Sometimes those closest to us want to keep us as victims. This can be because they are afraid we might hurt ourselves again should we ever venture out alone, or because they have an ulterior motive in retaining power over us, the poor helpless victim.

Many of us make the transition from victim to survivor at some point in our lives. Perhaps you have found your way out of overwork or workaholism, survived cancer or a life-threatening injury, domestic violence or sexual abuse, or you have lived through a natural disaster. If you're a survivor, how did you tap into your inner resources and strength to make the transition? How did you overcome your fear?

* Did you change your perspective on life and what's important?

* Did you focus on the feeling of relief that you got through it all?

* Did you celebrate being a survivor?

Survivors start to smile again, but there's still much to be learned before you can love or trust yourself or anyone else again. As a survivor, you develop greater resilience. You now have the tools you need for self-care, the resources that will serve to help you overcome future challenges and obstacles.

What remains now, if you're up for it, is to seek to become a thriver.

This means tackling those limiting self-beliefs and shifting your mindset to be more outward focused. It isn't easy. It takes time and perseverance and yes, you'll probably fall over a few times, grazing your knees in the process. Moving from just coping to being your true and authentic self is about choosing to direct and navigate your life's journey with joy, vulnerability and happiness.

Being a thriver allows you to let go of the emotional ties to the past. You haven't forgotten, but you're not stuck in your story. You're ready to trust yourself, to accept all your jiggly bits, to seek personal growth while taking responsibility and accountability for your actions.

Being a thriver encompasses everything: your life, work, health and relationships. It means living life on your terms free of blame or shame. How liberating is that!

A thriver is comfortable in their own skin. They flourish through having the confidence, self-awareness and empathy to know their limitations and vulnerabilities while stepping up to seek ways to make a positive difference and help others.

A thriver learns from and lets their past go.

Are you a survivor or thriver?

Thriver's mindset

I first came across the concept of a thriver's mindset through the work of Dr Dan Diamond, a medical practitioner based in the US who has specialised in coordinating disaster relief efforts for over thirty years.

Dr Dan cares deeply about people. You can sense it from the way he engages with them. His kindly manner, sharp wit and the twinkle in his eye belie a hidden strength of character and laser-sharp intelligence. He's the guy you definitely want to have around in the event of widespread tragedy or adversity.

It was his curiosity around the differences in human behaviour he observed in the face of tragedy following the aftermath of Hurricane Katrina in 2005 that led him to ask the question, 'What is it that enables a person to rise above victimhood, to stay fully engaged despite the many obstacles and challenges faced, to make a positive difference and leave a legacy?'

Perhaps you've noticed this difference too.

The Australian summer of 2019–20 began with bushfires on a scale never before experienced that left the nation reeling from the loss of life, livelihoods and property. The constant barrage of media updates including grim footage of fire and destruction, mass evacuations, stories of survival and death were overwhelming, exhausting and shocking.

Australians and others around the world responded. Donations of goods, food, clothing and blankets started pouring in. Money was pledged to the relief efforts. Offers of help came in all shapes and forms.

There were so many victims.

Most of us could scarcely imagine what it might feel like to lose everything but the clothes you're standing up in.

Yet, even early on, there was talk of starting over, of rebuilding. People affected, both directly and indirectly, expressed enormous gratitude towards the thousands of volunteer firefighters, army reservists and those who simply stepped in to help because they wanted to and could. There were numerous stories of courage and despair, of hope and loss.

A pattern started to emerge in the language being used:

+ The victims said, 'We've lost everything and need a lot of help fast'.

+ The survivors said, 'We've lost everything. We're so grateful for all the help we've received because it's going to be a long slow route to recovery, but we can do this'.

+ The thrivers said, 'We've lost everything, but we're still here. We're so grateful for all the help we've received, and now the community is coming together, and we're looking out for and supporting each other as we rebuild our lives'.

Dr Dan believes what differentiates victims, survivors and thrivers are the answers they give to the following two questions:

+ Will I choose to be powerful or powerless?

+ Will I act with purpose to give, or will I take?

Coming from a place of power and purpose will help you recover more quickly from even the most challenging of situations.

This is about:

+ your conscious choice of response

+ a willingness to accept your mistakes, failures or loss and being open to what you can do differently next time

+ acceptance of your situation, but knowing the past doesn't have to dictate your future.

This is the difference between what global mindset expert Professor Carol Dweck calls having a fixed or growth-oriented mindset.

A fixed mindset sees intelligence as innate. You're either smart or you're dumb. You've either got what it takes or you don't. You're either right or you're wrong. It's good or it's bad. There's no room for any shades of grey.

A growth mindset recognises how intelligence can be grown, that constructive feedback and failure can be useful to learn from, and that your effort and perseverance will guide you towards success.

Your choice of mindset matters

It matters to how you show up every day. It determines your attitude, your energy and your outcomes. Dweck believes it is our choice of mindset, not our intelligence or talent that determines our success.

Your state of mind comes fully emotionally charged, affecting you and everyone you come into contact with. Your mindset is not a single thing. It is a set of attitudes and beliefs shaped by experience and who you got to hang out with when very young. Yes, it's time to put your hands together and give thanks to Mum and Dad, who were complicit in shaping your mindset.

Being a choice and being shaped in this way means you can use your magnificent plastic brain to change your mind, rewiring neural circuits towards developing an outlook that will keep you happy and thriving.

As a composite being you're not stuck with a fixed or growth-oriented mindset. Much depends on what influences your state of mind at any point in time, including:

- **your emotions**. Are there things weighing on your mind? What concerns, worries and anxieties are you dealing with on a personal or work-related level?

- **your environment**. Are you in a place that makes you feel safe? Are there others around you who you know and trust, who are on your side, who get what you're trying to achieve and will look out for you?

- **your mental and physical wellbeing**. How well are you? Your level of fatigue, your internal resources of stress resilience, level of interest, general health, pain or hunger all play a part.

Creating a place of safety in a high-stress environment

There's a big difference between how we manage our mindset when operating in an environment that is calm, stable and predictable and when in a high-stress situation being shot at by snipers all around us. Like the time you're fending off those barbs of passive aggression from a colleague during a meeting. Or when you received that nasty email or social media comment. Or that time you received an urgent summons from your boss and had no idea why. Or when your world was tipped upside down by the threat of a global pandemic.

Under pressure we veer towards the negative and start assuming the worst. We engage in more 'what if' that frightens us.

Our sunny disposition can be severely put to the test when we're being shouted at, or we're dealing with someone we feel is being completely unreasonable or blaming us for their misfortune or are being relentlessly bombarded by negative media reports. Here the dimensions of power and purpose start to influence the different mindsets we experience every day.

If you're working super hard but finding it hard to maintain your motivation, it's easy to become despondent, and to start to feel disengaged from what used to give you that spark of passion and purpose. Drawing on your inner strength at this time can feel like a challenge. Making a decision founded on courage rather than fear requires what Dr Dan calls 'the choice of significance over safety'.

If the ship is sinking and the lifeboats are leaking, saving yourself and everyone else around you means asking yourself some questions:

+ What can I give here that will help everyone?
+ What other resources can I tap into that will make a difference?
+ What action am I going to take right now to make a start to bringing about the desired change?

When faced with adversity or a challenge which mindset do you adopt? Which question will help you adopt a thriver's or positive, growth-oriented mindset?

Changing your mindset

Cultivating a growth-oriented or thriver's mindset for greater success and happiness begins with a decision. It's yours to make.

Check your thoughts

Have you ever had one of those days where you wake up in a bad mood? The grey skies outside match your outlook. You grump into work with a frown and the expectation that the day won't go well. Guess what, it becomes a self-fulfilling prophecy.

On those days when you wake up in a good mood, not only does the sun seem brighter but you feel more capable, more confident and yes, you get more done. A positive state of mind helps you to acknowledge and accept the disappointments and failures you encounter along the way. Your thoughts create the feelings that lead to the behaviours that determine your outcomes. Checking your thoughts is the first step towards nurturing a more positive outlook.

Mind your language

If you find you're berating yourself with negative self-talk, nip it in the bud before it festers and becomes a self-defeating habit. Challenge yourself when you hear yourself thinking, *I'm hopeless at this. I was never going to win. Who am I kidding? This is never going to work!*

How can you reframe those statements to be kinder and encouraging to yourself? If I practise a bit more, I'll get better. I had the same chance as everyone else. I'll try again next year. I need to look at what I could do differently next time to get a different outcome.

This sort of self-encouragement is realistic optimism and is very different from 'just think positive' advice or blind faith, which is unhelpful. Albert Bandura reminds us it's the difference between thinking that success will come easily ('She'll be right') and that it will come with careful thought, planning and applied effort. If you expect a couple of roadblocks and obstacles on the way, you're better prepared and less likely to be caught off guard ('I didn't expect that to happen').

Whether you're on a diet, starting an exercise program to get fitter or signing up to take an online degree, anticipating that there will likely be a few hiccups better prepares you to deal with them effectively.

Set the intention

It only takes a moment to reset your thinking. Setting aside a couple of minutes to attune yourself to your thoughts and feelings at the beginning of the day equips you to make your choice and go from there. By regularly affirming your intention to have a good day, you can quickly shift from having an excess of not-so-great days to more great days at work.

Have you scheduled in that five minutes to reset?

Dial down the noise

Relish quiet and silence. Your day is probably full of noise; while some is no doubt enjoyable, constant exposure to the clamour of air-conditioners, traffic and your louder colleagues is a source of stress your brain does not habituate to. Over time continuous exposure to low-level ambient noise contributes to your stress. If this is already on the high side, you're at increased risk of developing a stress-related illness or mental health problem.

Yet getting comfortable with quiet can be a challenge, especially if you're not used to it. When I was small, our family lived on a busy main road. When we moved to a quieter street, none of us could sleep — the quiet kept us awake!

Quiet can be your friend, providing you with time to reflect, consider and reset.

Reduce negative inputs

It's good to stay informed about world events, but in the era of the 24/7 news cycle, when attention-grabbing headlines are repeated every hour, bad news provokes chronic anxiety, which in turn triggers the need for updates every five minutes.

Instead of relying on information from proven reliable sources, you start to read anything written by anyone with an opinion, whether or not they are qualified to share it. Far from alleviating your anxiety, repeated images and reports highlighting the dangers of scarcity, atrocity or disease further aggravate your internal stress response. The confusing and often contradictory information heightens your anxiety and draws you deeper into the social contagion.

Panic buying in times of crisis is one manifestation of social contagion, the entirely unnecessary toilet paper 'shortage' in the early days of the 2020 COVID-19 pandemic a perfect illustration. You're aware of events as they unfold and feel you're doing okay, but going down to your local supermarket you are shocked to find customers falling over each other to grab the last bulk packs of toilet paper. Looking around, you notice there are only a couple of jars of pasta sauce left on the shelves. You might not like pasta sauce, but you now put those two jars in your shopping basket 'just in case'.

By discriminating between useful and unreliable information, it becomes easier to manage any associated anxiety, to stay calm and focused, and to keep your mind set on what will best help you manage the situation.

Seek other perspectives

Your world view is unique to you and you alone. While hard to accept that not everyone shares your viewpoint (how can they not understand how your perspective is right — every time?), staying open and willing to hear alternative perspectives provides you with more options. It may not often change your view, but sometimes it might, and it will help you to understand why others think differently.

Ditch perfectionism

Perfectionism sucks, because it's unattainable. The more we seek perfection, the harder we make things for ourselves and the more unhappy we become. There is beauty in imperfection, when we permit ourselves to see it.

Kintsugi or Kintsukuroi is the Japanese art of repairing broken pots using lacquer mixed with precious metals such as gold or silver, transforming what was broken into something even more beautiful than it was in its original form.

The philosophy of embracing our flaws and imperfections can help us to overcome the pain of a broken relationship, a failed business, or the struggle associated with being an entrepreneur or single parent.

Abandon victimhood

Staying the victim means always being weighed down by the heavy mantle of guilt and shame. It's normal to grieve a loss, but the victim remains stuck, unable to let go of all the unfairness and injustice, so unable to heal.

Squeeze out the impostor

It's getting harder to find anyone not afflicted to some degree by impostordom. Research suggests 70 per cent of us experience it at some point in our lives, while for some it's taken up residence as a permanent unwelcome squatter. No matter our title, achievements and awards, that niggling feeling of self-doubt encourages flaws, inadequacies and ugly self-talk, downplaying our hard efforts as a fluke or error. It's time to stand tall and call out the negative self-talk for what it is, and accept 'we did okay' and feel good about it.

Surround yourselves with people who inspire you

Having more positive and optimistic people around you provides a useful reality check and helps minimise catastrophic thinking, especially important in those times when you're in a bit of a funk and in desperate need of inspiration.

Get out of the armchair of comfort

Change can be scary, overwhelming and tiring. But without change we do not grow, and without growth we fail to adapt and evolve. Challenging the status quo, stepping out of your comfort zone, is going to be uncomfortable, and yes it can get messy and possibly not deliver what you hoped for. But that's okay because it shows you tried and if you don't try there's little hope of achieving your dreams. So get comfy with the discomfort of doing something that scares you a little, because you know it has the potential to make a positive difference.

A stretch goal is energising and motivating. It could be the thing that radically changes your life for the better. How great is it going to feel when you succeed?

Be the change and love it. Because as Abraham Maslow said, 'One can choose to go back toward safety or forward toward growth. Growth must be chosen again and again; fear must be overcome again and again'.

Your prescription for a thriver's mindset

- Believe in your capacity and potential to bring about positive change.
- Choose to challenge those self-limiting beliefs.
- Take action, however small, to start you off.
- Celebrate all your wins and fails.
- Let go of the need to be in control of everything.
- Abandon the need for perfection.
- Live as a thriver with passion, love and gratitude.
- Maintain a realistic optimism.
- Choose to work with other thrivers.
- Choose abundance over scarcity, courage over fear.

Part III

Thriving

Opening up the throttle to fully thrive

The secret of getting ahead is getting started. The secret of getting started is breaking down your complex overwhelming tasks into small manageable tasks, and then starting on the first one.
Mark Twain

Derived from the Old Norse *thrifta*, meaning to grasp or grab hold of, whether you have thrived, throve or thriven, thriving today indicates that you're doing well and feeling good about yourself and your life. *Merriam-Webster*'s definition is to 'grow vigorously, flourish', conveying the sense of a state that can be nurtured like a plant with plenty of food, water and sunlight.

So how do we do this? The first step is to remember you are not a machine; you are human, with basic physiological and psychological limitations. Ignore them at your peril. Our fast-paced, 24/7 world places unrealistic expectations on all of us. Our workplaces often value productivity over humanity. So it's up to us, to you, to draw some boundaries and optimise your own physical and psychological needs. By making lifestyle choices that support you, you can bring the healthiest and best version of yourself to everything you do.

 Self-care is never selfish; it's essential to being your best self.

Being your best self means you have more to offer, both at work and at home. In the following chapters we will be looking at six essential elements of your lifestyle aspects that support you and contribute to creating the healthiest version of you:

1. rest and recovery

2. enough sleep

3. healthy eating

4. regular exercise

5. music and dance

6. time in nature.

You might have some of these in hand, which is fantastic (you can skip those chapters, or read them to validate your great choices so far), but the key is to have them ALL in hand. For example, you might have a great diet and get plenty of exercise, but if you're stressed out of your brain and not sleeping then your wellbeing is far from complete.

The choices we make lead to the behaviours we develop. Our habits are often deeply entrenched from years of practice, which can make them very difficult to change. In the final part of the book I'll be sharing more around the 'how' of behavioural change and how to set yourself up for greater success.

Thriving is about how well we adapt to change and how well we implement behaviours that keep us at our best by creating supportive patterns of thinking and habits and treating ourselves as human beings rather than machines.

Now it's time to thrive.

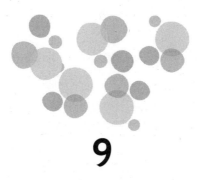

9

Rest and recovery – the key to resilience

It is really wonderful how much resilience there is in human nature. Let any obstructing cause, no matter what, be removed in any way, even by death, and we fly back to first principles of hope and enjoyment.
Bram Stoker, *Dracula*

A couple of years ago I was invited to run a workshop on resilience for a Sydney-based engineering company. The challenge was that their top-performing managers, a highly skilled, dedicated and close-knit group, were failing. Their performance was slipping, but what worried the leadership team most was the impact this was having on their family life. Relationships were breaking down, families being torn apart by divorce, and the atmosphere at work was one of increasing frustration and unhappiness.

The reason? They had forgotten how to switch off.

That small switch — you know, the one that allows you to stop thinking about work, that denies you access to your work emails or permission to spend your whole weekend working. You put that automated message on your phone advising your working hours and that you'll get back to the caller. Later.

Does your commitment, love for what you do or sense of duty keep you at work longer than needed? Is there an expectation or unwritten ground rule that you'll always stay late and get in early? If you're a small business owner or entrepreneur, do you ever wonder how the idea of being your own boss somehow translated into missing out on the rest of your life, of having to call your partner to say sorry you'll be home late (again) or to make another excuse not to join your friends for a night out?

You spend more than one-third of your life at work and while doing work that you enjoy is highly rewarding and fulfilling, this shouldn't be at the expense of the other aspects of your life that enable you to thrive and be happy.

In the digital age, when resources are not always available, support is thin on the ground and the expectation is to keep doing more with less, it's all too common to think the only way forward is to keep grinding away, nose down, tail up.

We are encouraged to 'toughen up', 'show some grit' and 'suck it up, Princess'. But resilience doesn't work this way. It's not just endurance and pain. Which is why thrivers understand the key to resilience is to include time every day for rest and recovery.

 Sustainable resilience includes sufficient down time for rest and recovery.

Rest and recovery bolsters resilience and mental wellbeing

Is it possible to be a successful top performer and still have the time and energy to feel fulfilled and happy in other aspects of your life? Absolutely it is. You can have it all by addressing your physiological and psychological needs to optimise your wellbeing and keep you at the top of your game.

 Thriving starts by remembering you are human.

What gets us into trouble is when we take those shortcuts, such as believing it's possible to get by on less sleep, ignoring our rising stress levels and treating ourselves as machine not human.

Sorry to be the bearer of bad news, but you're not a superhero, even if you've got the pyjama set from Peter Alexander. Let's get real and take a look at what the science says about the benefits of taking a mental break.

The brainy benefits of rest

If your job entails constantly absorbing new information, handling vast swathes of data and especially working with a screen for many hours at a time, you'll know how exhausting it can be. Even unlimited enthusiasm isn't enough to confound the mental fatigue that soon slips in uninvited.

Research has confirmed that our performance improves when we take frequent short breaks. In one study a group of healthy volunteers were shown a series of numbers on a screen then asked to type those numbers as many times as possible in 10 seconds using their left hand before taking a 10-second break, and repeating the process 35 times while their brain waves were monitored.

Yes, absolutely riveting stuff. Not. What they found, though, was that even a tiny rest like this boosted performance. *Have you ever found taking a break useful for refreshing your attention and focus for the task at hand?*

If you're having difficulty retaining even a fraction of the information you're exposed to every day, fret not. So does everybody else. You can help your brain to filter out and save the most relevant details by:

- making the information as appealing as possible (yes, it certainly helps if you're interested in what you're doing)

- taking a mental break to allow the subconscious part of your brain to register the dopamine reward of learning and stimulate memory consolidation.

The moral of the story is that sleep *and* rest are vital for learning and memory.

 ## Rest enhances memory consolidation and learning.

It has long been thought that keeping our brain fully occupied is the way to boost productivity, but science has shown that relying on unrelenting focused thought is mentally taxing and quickly leads to brain fog and mental fatigue.

By occasionally uncoupling from focus to run on idle, the brain automatically switches to the default mode network (DMN), one of five resting state networks that provide the brain with vital down time:

- to make sense of what we have learned

- to allow us to switch to autopilot once we have learned a task, such as driving

- for self-reflection

- for exercising our imagination

◆ to absorb how we respond to what we consider beautiful

◆ to stimulate creativity through engaging the DMN, the salience network and the executive network.

The switch is automatic and swift, occurring in the blink of an eye. Your DMN is briefly activated with each blink and turned off again when the eye reopens. *Did you ever wonder why we sometimes choose to think with our eyes closed?*

If we keep pushing ourselves beyond our physiological limits, we put ourselves at greater risk of overtraining and burnout. Forget the old adage of practice makes perfect. This is only true if you engage in deliberate practice. Psychologist Anders Ericsson examined the practice habits of talented individuals at the pinnacle of their powers. Whether musician, athlete or writer, these elite performers typically don't practise for more than four hours a day, and they prefer to start training early in the morning when they are mentally and physically fresh.

Which is why, where possible, it's best to schedule your most cognitively demanding work for early in the day, keeping less mentally taxing work such as meetings for the afternoon. Adopting this smarter approach you work less, but in a more productive way, to achieve more.

It's all in the CLM

When you've got too much on your mental plate, it's time to call in the cognitive load management team. Do you ever take time out to defrag and destress? Have you ever taken advantage of your company's policy permitting mental health days? While 'chucking a sickie' is often frowned on, if stress is getting the better of you taking time out for your mental health can be a useful stopgap measure to lower the risk of blowing your head gasket.

Of course, this doesn't fix the underlying problem if chronic overwork, sleep deprivation, anxiety and/or depression are the cause. These problems require a longer term strategy to resolve, but taking the occasional mental health day is a good place to start.

Taking time off after completing a major project is helpful too. If you and your team have spent weeks burning the candle at both ends, pulling all-nighters, it benefits your physical and mental wellbeing to take some well-deserved time off to rest. Does your workplace encourage rest to keep you energised and refreshed?

Rest allows the body and mind to reset and refresh following an intense period of mental or physical work.

Cited as an essential for our new working era, CLM is about recognising your mental load limits — how much your brain can realistically handle before overloading the executive suite of higher order thinking and running the risk of poor judgement, bad decision making, big mistakes and expanding mental fatigue.

Inserting a couple of short brain breaks in your day helps you to restore your attention and cognitive performance and impress others with your ability to stay alert even when faced with back-to-back meetings all day.

So schedule a lunch break, and take it. Yes, a novel idea, I know. But did you know at least half the Australian workforce fail to take a lunchbreak every day? Worse still is to eat while remaining chained to your desk. If you knew the bacterial count on your keyboard, you'd know it would be more hygienic to eat off the bathroom floor.

Eating 'al desko' is not a break, it's a health hazard!

Other natural breaks include the 10- or 15-minute mid-morning and mid-afternoon pauses, previously known as tea breaks. It's time to bring these civilised institutions back into fashion. Your choice of beverage is irrelevant. Far more important is allowing yourself that short, unfocused breathing space in which to rest, giving your subconscious the consolidation time it needs.

Taking a technology break

Early in 2020 hubby and I booked a holiday at a place where there was no internet access or mobile phone coverage. While we hadn't specifically booked a digital detox, the impact of not being able to check on emails (in case something important cropped up), not listening to yet more doom and gloom on the world news, and not worrying about what was happening elsewhere felt liberating. By day three I'd stopped wearing my watch and felt strangely calm. I realised I hadn't felt so relaxed and unfettered by stress and work for a very long time.

Studies have shown how taking even a short break from our technology starts to lower stress levels and blood pressure, generating a greater sense of calm and wellbeing. Many of us are engaged with our screens for more than ten hours a day. How does technology affect you? If you've ever caught yourself picking up your phone and scrolling to see if there are any incoming messages since you last checked *five minutes ago*, or it's become your way of filling in time whenever you have a couple of minutes to spare, putting some boundaries around your technology use can be a helpful way of improving your physical, emotional and mental wellbeing.

Screen-Free Week is held each year around late April or early May as a reminder to take a fresh look at our relationship with our electronic media. But you don't have to wait till then to gain the benefits of switching off, which include:

- **being more in the present moment.** You're back 'in real time'

- **more conversation.** Instead of sitting next to friends and colleagues while glued to your mobile device, you can enjoy meaningful conversations and deepen connection

- **increasing your ability to pay attention and stay on task.** The more your attention is fragmented, the more difficult it becomes to focus on anything well

- **better sleep.** Rather than keeping your brain hyperstimulated, your natural sleep inducers get a chance to weave their magic.

If the thought of switching off is making you twitchy, take it slowly. Try 20 minutes as a starter when you know you don't need to be on your phone, such as during mealtimes, in the bathroom or when having sex. Yes, some things are no longer sacred. Sigh. Be accountable for your own actions. There are apps available to tell you how much time you've spent online. Shocked? Okay, it's time to reach for the off button more often.

Reconsider your choice of social media channels. Switch off notifications or remove a channel altogether. If Facebook frustrates you, it could be time to say *sayonara* and leave it behind you.

 If social media is making you twitchy, it's time to switch off.

Mental work is tiring

Too much mental activity can wear you out. Your brain, like any other part of your body, if overtaxed, will suffer from fatigue in the same way an athlete gets sore muscles if they overtrain.

Does this mean you should stop thinking? Heck no. But if you have a tendency to worry or overthink, it's especially important for you to build in some strategies to minimise the potential impact.

One theory as to why thinking hard is tiring relates to the brain chemical called adenosine (you'll be hearing more about this substance later in the book). Adenosine is produced in increasing amounts over the course of the day to prepare us for sleep.

Thinking hard burns a lot of mental energy, specifically glucose, and especially in those brain areas associated with demanding mental processing such as the prefrontal cortex and anterior cingulate cortex. Running out of mental fuel triggers a rise in adenosine levels, which in turn blocks the effects of dopamine, the neurotransmitter involved in motivation and reward. Which explains why at the end of the day, when you've run out of mental juice, you feel exhausted and in no state to carry on working.

It's only during sleep that the adenosine is flushed out of your brain so you wake up in the morning feeling bright eyed and bushy tailed. Being sleep deprived aggravates the problem because the higher levels of adenosine are now working to persuade you to go to bed.

If fatigue ever leads you to delay making a difficult decision, that's probably not a bad thing. In the Israeli Parole Judges Study, it was found that judges presiding over parole cases were more lenient — that is, more likely to grant parole — when feeling fresh and alert after taking a lunchbreak. *Note to self: if ever up before a parole board hearing, try to arrange it that your application is first on the list, or the one immediately after lunch.*

Our mental fatigue also explains our love of coffee as a pick-me-up to enhance mental alertness, as we will examine in a later chapter.

Mental fatigue impairs physical performance

If your job is cognitively demanding, your risk of having an accident or work-related mishap rises when you're feeling tired because fatigue impairs our physical performance.

Researchers from Wales have shown how watching a 90-minute documentary on a computer screen then getting onto an exercise bike for a time-to-exhaustion test made the physical part of the test feel harder so they gave up sooner, compared with another group who didn't watch the documentary first.

Not sure how this relates to you? Okay, let's look at it another way. When you have sat beavering away on your computer for 90 minutes, the level of fatigue created is equivalent to jumping on and off a 35 cm box 100 times! How do your legs feel now?

Managing your cognitive load is about recognising your own mental and physical limits and working within safe boundaries.

Which rest is best?

Rest takes different forms. Why not mix and match to find your ideal combination?

The mini rest: for daily consumption

It's easy to discount the value of a mini rest, but taking a couple of minutes out of your day to pause and breathe can make a mountain of difference to your energy level, productivity and happiness. The mini rest is super exclusive because this is *yours only* to savour and enjoy. Hurrah!

Start by scheduling in some mini brain breaks into your day.

If your day is full of back-to-back meetings, appointments and stuff-that-has-to-be-completed-by-the-end-of-the-day-or-I'm-in-big-trouble, block your time into chunks of focused work separated by two or three intervals of 5–10 minutes of unfocused non-thinking time. And no, this is definitely *not* the time to check your social media.

Why not drink some water, top up your coffee cup or get up for a stretch? Standing up for two or three minutes gives your body and brain a breather, boosts attention and is a great mini refresher. Or indulge in a mini day-dream to fire up your imagination and creativity. We're not designed for long-term focus, so loosen those attention straps and take a break.

The midi rest: extending the mini

A midi rest lasts between 15 and 20 minutes. This could be your chance to escape the office and get some fresh air and sunshine, go for a short walk or jog, catch up with a friend, meditate, listen to some music or take a power nap. Or try a technology-free recess, turning your mobile to silent and closing your laptop to alleviate stress and reduce the perception of time passing too quickly.

The major rest: advance bookings are being taken now

Life is often one big, messy, shambolic blur. If you've been relying on strategies that involve keeping a tight control on things using some well-thumbed obsessive-compulsive techniques or Marie Kondo program, adhering too rigidly to your own rules can be counterproductive and serve only to heighten stress and muscle tension. It's time to take time out for yours truly.

Yes, you. This is your 'me time'. Let go. Give someone else a turn at the wheel for a change. That's what great leaders do: they provide others with the opportunity to learn how to steer the boat, because how else can they gain the experience necessary to navigate dangerous waters full of submerged obstacles and predators with sharp pointy teeth?

Making yourself redundant because you have allowed others to practise taking their trainer wheels off frees you up to be absent, confident in the knowledge that all will be well until your return.

Take a holiday—you've earned it. Not only that, but you'll come back feeling brighter, more energised and inspired to do more. *How has taking leave helped you deal with your heavy workload, manage the disruption of change and deal with all of life's nuances and challenges?*

With 55 per cent of Australians failing to take their scheduled annual leave, what does your rest planner look like? The things to include during a major rest are those that give you joy. These might include music, trekking, cooking, exercising, socialising, sleeping, travelling, or spending time with your partner and family.

Planning ahead and scheduling in that longer break ensures that it happens and gives you something to look forward to. How many sleeps to your next holiday?

Your prescription for rest and recovery

- Schedule in down time for a mini, midi or major break. No negotiation permitted!

- Factor in enough down time for recovery to reduce stress by engaging in those activities (such as exercise, music or massage) that give you pleasure and take your mind off your worries.

- If work is going crazy and you're currently racking up a lot of overtime, check there is an expiry date on the project, schedule in down time for when it is completed, and in the meantime ensure you're getting enough sleep and taking mini breaks across your day.

- Recognise when you're reaching your cognitive limit and press the pause button. Pushing through to complete an assignment when you're mentally fatigued will cost you more in the long run, causing more mistakes and poorer decision making.

- Less can be more. Factoring in time for sleep, exercise, meditation and rest, while consuming time, repays you with clearer thinking and less stress, so you're more effective and productive in the time available.

- Allocate time for catch-ups. Socialising helps to keep things in perspective. Sharing stories and experiences reminds us we all struggle sometimes. Our resilience is strengthened and supported by knowing we're not alone.

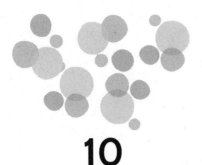

10

Sleep – not just for the wicked

Sleep is non-negotiable. Period. It's the foundation of good health and essential to our survival.

J.B.

As a junior doctor working in the NHS in the UK in the eighties, I was required to be 'on call' in addition to working my regular Monday to Friday daytime hours. This could mean anything from every fifth night (pure luxury) to every second (pure hell).

While working at what would today be called an aged care hospital in South London (an old workhouse built in 1832, it was later converted into a geriatric infirmary), I drew the short straw to cover a public holiday weekend, which meant I was the on-call duty medical officer from Friday morning until Tuesday afternoon and the only doctor physically present in the hospital from Friday evening onwards. Not only that, but my Senior Registrar was busy studying for his physician's exams and had made it perfectly clear he didn't want to be called in except in an extreme emergency.

It was a really busy weekend. By Sunday evening I had been able to snatch only a few hours' sleep and was finding it increasingly hard to stay awake. My eyes ached with fatigue.

Monday was a complete blur but a little quieter, so after doing my late-night round at around 10.30 pm I slunk off to the on-call room, a small space with a single bed, bedside cabinet, small lamp and hand basin, to grab a couple of hours' shuteye.

I was jerked out of a restless sleep when my pager went off. A patient had died and I was required to certify death so the body could be moved from the ward to the morgue.

There was one small problem. In my befuddled, sleep-deprived state I hadn't taken note of which ward had called, and the pager shed no light on where the call had come from. So there was only one thing to do: I went from ward to ward asking if they had just lost a patient.

Curiously none of them said they had.

Now thoroughly mystified, but still convinced a patient had died, I went off to the morgue to double check a new body hadn't been recently delivered.

No one had died that night. Insufficient sleep had not only clouded my judgement but led to the creation of a false memory.

The call was a figment of my imagination.

How does lack of sleep affect you? Have you ever had one of those moments when you were convinced you'd sent that email, paid that bill or called that client, only to find it was your brain playing tricks on you — again!

Have you ever found yourself a bit tetchy, irritable and unlovable because you're just so darn tired? And what about that time when you'd pulled an all-nighter, desperate to meet that deadline, and realised the moment you pressed Send that there was a glaring error on the first page?

Lack of sleep does us no good and yet getting enough seems like a growing challenge.

The secrets of sleep

Sleep scientists have discovered much more about its secrets — why we, along with virtually every other creature on this planet, need sleep, its different functions and what happens to us when we are chronically denied it.

Sleep is much more than getting some rest. During sleep your brain is incredibly active sorting out all the incoming information accumulated during the day, determining what needs to be kept for long-term storage and starting the process of consolidating long-term memory, loosening synaptic connections (so you forget information no longer needed) to free up more space for new memory, regulating your emotions, and taking out the trash the brain has accumulated during the day.

Sleep is highly complex. Sleep disruption, whether or not it is 'intentional' (such as through shift work), has a significant impact on our ability to feel refreshed and restored in the morning. Sleep plays an important role in regulating a range of different genes and endocrine systems that contribute to our mood, happiness, wellbeing and relationships.

 Getting enough sleep is essential to your complete health and wellbeing.

It's time for a sleep party: get into the rhythm

Sleep is regulated by two systems. The homeostatic sleep drive tracks how long you've been awake. The longer your period of wakefulness, the stronger the drive to find a nice comfy bed. You can think of it as a manager balancing your sleep and wakefulness. The drive to sleep is highest between 2 and 4 am and again in the early afternoon around 1 to 3 pm, perfect for that post-prandial, 20-minute power nap.

Maybe you've noticed too how when you're sleep deprived that urge to sleep becomes increasingly hard to resist no matter how many matchsticks you use to keep your eyes prised open. You'll also fall into a longer, deeper sleep when in this state.

What keeps you awake for around 16 hours each day is determined by your internal circadian biological clock, which regulates a number of what are called circadian rhythms. It's controlled by the suprachiasmatic nucleus (SCN), which responds to light, telling us to stay awake, and prevents the release of melatonin, the hormone produced at night that promotes sleep. As darkness falls, melatonin levels rise and the signal is now it's time to sleep.

Determining the best time to go to bed requires two valuable pieces of information:

- **how much sleep you need**. While most of us require around eight hours, we are all unique. Whether you function best on nine hours or seven doesn't matter. Understanding what works best for you does. Remember, too, this is time spent sleeping, which may be very different from the total time spent in bed.

- **what time you need to be up in the morning**. Say you function best on eight hours' sleep and need to be up at 6.30 am. Ideally this will mean lights out at between 10.15 and 10.30 pm, depending how long it takes you to fall asleep.

The sleep calculator at startsleeping.org goes one step further by taking into consideration your age and the total number of sleep cycles you will complete in that time frame.

One of the best ways to get into the habit of going to bed at the ideal time, rather than being dictated to by the end of the work you're doing or the Netflix series you're binge watching, is to set an alarm clock for bedtime.

If you're a night owl who finds it hard to go to bed early or wake up in good time there are a number of tech gadgets you can turn to for help. For example, consider trying a natural light alarm clock set at an intensity of 200 Lux that helps you to wake feeling refreshed. This can be helpful if you're living in an area where dawn doesn't break until later in the morning in the winter months. Some come with a sunset function too, with dimming sunset colours (nice!) and the option of appropriate soothing sounds.

Why we choose to sleep less

Sometimes I wake up a little grumpy,
and sometimes I let him sleep in.
Anon

If you've ever had to live with a grumpy, sleep-deprived two-year-old, you know how important it is to get enough sleep. And yet we often choose to cut back on our quota:

- because we're busy and insist on squeezing more stuff into our work day
- because we think we can train ourselves to get by with less
- because it makes us feel in some way superior to other mere mortals.

The trouble is this is wrong on every count.

Unless you are a giraffe who manages perfectly well on two hours' sleep a night (mostly taken as a series of five-minute giraffe naps) or a dolphin with the rather nifty ability to adopt uni-hemispheric sleep to ensure you stay safe from unwelcome marine predators, or you are genuinely the proud owner of the so-called short sleep gene, like the rest of us you'll need somewhere between seven and nine hours of good-quality uninterrupted sleep to function at your best.

Surely we can train ourselves to do with less

I get that spending one-third of your life asleep might seem like a waste of time, but the nocturnal activities of your brain have been demonstrated to be vital to your daily functioning, and your mental and physical health, including your cognition and weight.

You've probably heard that certain individuals, such as Margaret Thatcher, Winston Churchill, Elon Musk and Donald Trump, reportedly need or needed only four to six hours' sleep. Three genes associated with being a short sleeper have now been identified, but unless you've had the genetic profiling done to prove it, I'm sorry to break it to you but any belief that you are a member of this select club is nothing short of delusional.

The world's largest sleep study, conducted in Ontario, Canada, looked at the sleeping habits of more than 10 000 people from around the world to see if geographical location and habitat made a difference.

They didn't, but what they did find was that:

1. too much sleep is as bad as too little, putting you at greater risk of heart attack or stroke. Please don't fret; the number of people who truly sleep too much regularly is very small

2. 50 per cent of those surveyed were getting less than the recommended amount — typically around 6.3 hours — indicating that an enormous number of people are chronically sleep deprived. The worst thing about this, beyond increasing their risk of making mistakes, losing their cool, or losing concentration behind the wheel and causing an accident, is that they lose sight of just how tired they are.

Getting enough sleep reduces your risk of cardiovascular disease because it protects against atherosclerosis, or hardening of the arteries, and regulates the production of inflammatory cells in the bone marrow through the production of a hormone called hypocretin. One Japanese study linked less than six hours' sleep to a 500 per cent increase in risk of heart attack compared with those who slept as long as they needed to.

If you were looking for a reason for putting a higher value on sleep, this is a good place to start:

 Sleep deprivation increases your risk of, and death from, heart disease by 45 per cent.

That is not a typo.

It can also make you fat!

Sleep deprivation is terrible for your waistline

Sleep deprivation upsets a number of hormones. For starters it raises cortisol levels, which makes your cells more resistant to insulin, the hormone that drives sugar out of the bloodstream to where it needs to be used for energy. Other hormones are affected, including thyroid-stimulating hormone and testosterone (yes ladies, we have testosterone too, just less than men), further altering insulin sensitivity and resulting in higher blood sugar levels. This puts you at increased risk of developing type 2 diabetes. The waistline effect comes from the increase in ghrelin, the hormone that drives us to eat because we're hungry and the lowering of leptin, which tells us we're full thanks, it's time now to stop eating and start using up energy.

When Jan came to see me at the surgery, she was not happy. 'Tell me,' she pleaded, 'why is it that despite spending an hour and a half at the gym every day and starving myself on my current diet, the scales have not moved one jot over the past six weeks?' What Jan hadn't factored in was how her stressful job and poor sleeping patterns were conspiring against her desire to shift a couple of kilos.

Feeling groggy from lack of sleep doesn't just affect your level of attention; it dulls your brain's ability to make good decisions and control your impulses. If sleep is consistently missing in action, your body seeks out a metabolic boost because you are more susceptible to craving carbohydrate-rich foods, especially in the afternoon and at night, leading you to consume an average additional 300 calories per day. And when tired, it's harder to find the motivation to exercise.

Even one bad night's sleep is enough to drive you to eat more the following day.

Eve Van Cauter, director of the Sleep, Metabolism and Health Center at the University of Chicago, comments, 'Our body is not wired for sleep deprivation. The human is the only mammal that does this'.

 Being sleep deprived drives us to eat more.

The further bad news is that trying to catch up on sleep on the weekend can work against you. Research published in *Current Biology* shows that this practice won't stop the weight gain associated with sleep deprivation during the week. And research from the University of Colorado found that one week of insufficient sleep (around five hours a night) was enough to lead to a weight gain of two pounds (0.9 kilos). Too little sleep also affects our fat cells, reducing their ability to respond to the insulin needed to regulate our blood sugar and energy use, putting us at greater risk of weight gain and type 2 diabetes.

No wonder Jan wasn't happy.

I introduced her to some techniques for lowering her stress and increasing her sleep time, and she came back six weeks later in triumph. Her cravings for fat- and sugar-laden foods were reduced, she was feeling more energetic — and yes, she'd finally lost some weight.

A world full of zombies

If it's been a while since you last slept well, your normal sleep pattern (which isn't) has become so entrenched it's hard to remember what it feels like to sleep without waking during the night as your mind whirls from too much to worry about, think about and plan. Or your kids wake you up, your partner snores, or the dog is taking up most of the bed space, causing you to overheat.

How much sleep you need is personal. If you can wake up at the appropriate time feeling alert and refreshed without having to hit the snooze button three times, you've had enough sleep. The 7–9 hours is a guide, not an absolute rule.

Your sleep needs may differ from your partner's, so if you both have to get up at the same time your going-to-bed time may need to vary slightly.

During my Gap Year I slept. A lot. Catching up on years of sleep deprivation as part of the healing process. I have since developed a much healthier attitude towards sleep, recognising it as a wonderful means of achieving better emotional regulation and a more positive mood, with the bonus of smarter thinking.

Too tired to think?

Being overtired when at work is like being stuck on the highway to hell. You're just not functioning properly and are unable to shift your brain out of neutral.

The cognitive effect of sleep deprivation is a reduction in attention and working memory, meaning you're slower at processing new information. If being drunk at work isn't tolerated, the salient question is why we stay at work when we're exhausted, because going without sleep when pulling an all-nighter has the same effect on your thinking as registering a 0.05 blood alcohol reading.

Too tired to drive?

The first insight to leave the building when we're chronically tired is recognising just how tired we really are. So when driving tired we usually fail to do the sensible thing, which is to pull over and take a break. Instead we rationalise our stupidity: *It's not far now. I can stay awake if I wind the window down to let in some cold air, and play some loud music.* The only thing that has changed is that you now have a cold ear and are at risk of future hearing loss. You are still tired, and still a menace on the road at risk of causing an accident. We've got the message about not drinking and driving. Now we've got to understand not to drive tired.

I mentioned that dolphins are capable of uni-hemispheric sleep, enabling them to shut down one side of their brain while keeping the other side alert for predators. Unfortunately, we don't have an app for this. What our brain does do is shut down for a microsleep or turn off a group of neurons to allow them to rest. This is your brain's desperate attempt to avoid a total power cut by shutting down smaller circuits.

That's nifty, but not so great if you're asleep at the wheel. Microsleeps can last from a fraction of a second to several seconds, and on the road they're potentially deadly. The thing about microsleeps is that you may not even be aware they're happening, but hey you just missed that red light and failed to allow for the sharp bend in the road there.

Vulnerability to microsleeps rises among shift workers, and those who suffer from chronic sleep deprivation, insomnia or sleep apnoea. Doctors take note. Your superpowers do not cover you for this risk.

 Microsleeps are potentially deadly.

Stuck in the negative

Getting enough sleep helps your brain to keep your emotions in check, because a rested brain has lower cortisol levels and the prefrontal cortex, the part of your brain used for higher-order thinking is better able to apply the brakes as needed to dampen down the activity of the amygdala, the part of the brain that generates and interprets emotions if it's getting a little frisky and veering towards greater negativity bias.

Flash floods of tears and wildly unpredictable reactions can be indications of a poor night's sleep. Worrying over what went wrong can keep you in that dark space. And your unending self-criticism keeps you feeling bad. You're more at risk of being impulsive, showing poor judgement and making bad decisions.

Worse still, if you've had a horrible day, or a series of horrible days, sleep deprivation undermines the way your brain would normally process those experiences to help you make better sense of what happened and deal with the memories in a more helpful way. This can lead to the accumulation of a pile of unresolved and possibly painful memories. If these get stuck on continual replay, this can put you at greater risk of mood disorders such as anxiety and depression.

Lack of sleep means the amygdala gets more trigger-happy, firing off more intense emotions, both good and bad. It's not just the negative you need to be mindful of. Any slightly maniacal reaction can be a response to sleep deprivation.

If you're a natural worrier, sleep deprivation can add to your anxiety about the future. Getting stuck in all those 'what ifs' and uncertainties can aggravate your sleeping disorder and cause your anxiety levels to rise further.

If sleep is a premium you'd gladly pay more for, how is your lack of sleep currently impacting your emotional wellbeing?

 ### Lack of sleep can accentuate anxiety.

Lack of sleep isn't good for your relationships

Sleeping poorly has been shown to reduce our level of appreciation or gratitude towards our partners. Feeling good about each other starts by showing our appreciation and gratitude in simple ways, like saying 'thank you'. No one likes being taken for granted. If you aren't sleeping well, you'll tend to become a tad more selfish and self-focused, less empathetic and poorer at picking up emotional cues, all of which can prevent you from being the caring partner you normally are.

If both of you are sleep deprived, look out! This could herald the start of more arguments and less willingness to compromise on both sides.

 ### Lack of sleep is kryptonite to relationships.

Jet lag anyone?

If your work requires air travel across different time zones, you'll know just how awful being jetlagged makes you feel. You've got a presentation to deliver, but your brain tells you it's really still 3 o'clock in the morning and it's not prepared to log on that early to help you out.

There's a world of difference between flying west or east. Perhaps you've noticed travelling eastwards across multiple time zones is much harder for your system to adjust to. It's thought it's because it's harder to advance than delay the body's internal clock. For example, when flying west from Australia to Europe, arriving in the early morning, it doesn't feel too hard extending your day despite the eight- or nine-hour time difference. Flying from Europe to Australia, you're covering the same number of time zones but how often do you find you're dog tired but your brain won't allow you to sleep through those first couple of nights? Recovery time from jet lag can be doubled when flying east, depending on your individual sensitivity to time zone change.

Can jet lag be avoided? According to the 2020 Wellness Trends from the Global Wellness Summit the answer is yes.

Regular travellers commonly resort to melatonin pills (helpful), sedative drugs (not so great) or alcohol (a known sleep killer). A better option may be one of the new light travel apps such as Timeshifter, which takes into account your normal sleep pattern, whether you use melatonin and your itinerary to advise you when best to sleep or stay awake. This may conflict what the cabin crew would like you to do, but don't be put off. You might be the only person unaffected by jet lag on disembarking.

I'll be trying this out on my next trip to Europe and will let you know how I go.

Become the master of your busy brain

There's nothing more frustrating than falling into bed, exhausted from the day. Initially you fall asleep, but soon you're awake again because your brain has just nudged you to get into your party gear because there's a mega all-night thinking party raging in your head.

When the neighbours are playing their music too loud at 2 am, you can hope to get their attention and persuade them to turn the noise down. Sadly, it's really hard to achieve the same outcome with your own brain.

A common reason this can become an annoying habit that our brain falls into is that we've failed to provide enough down time during the day for our mind to consolidate all those thoughts and ideas, to arrive at a decision on what needs to be done next — and on and on.

Busy Brain Syndrome is a condition I've seen many times, especially in smart, savvy, self-driven, highly motivated individuals who are keen to make their mark, people whose brains operate continuously at warp .speed six, and in their determination to keep thinking at any cost, forget that taking time off during the day for *not* thinking is essential for a good night's refreshing sleep.

Every night as you travel through the 90- to 120-minute sleep cycles you spend time in light sleep, deep sleep and REM sleep. Each type of sleep matters for optimal health and functioning but it's the amount of time spent in deep sleep that is essential to waking up fresh as a daisy with a fully rested and refreshed brain.

Overbusy brains that think too much (you'll know if you fall into the overthinking category) benefit from learning how to slip in a couple of brain breaks during the day, a 10- to 20-minute mental pause when you switch off from heavy-lifting, higher-order-focused thinking and allow yourself time to enter the default mode.

Among the multiple intrinsic rhythms that feature in our life the ultradian rhythm is the one that regulates energy flow. Contrary to popular belief we are not designed for long-term focused thought, because it consumes too much of our precious mental energy of which we have only a limited daily supply.

Taking a brain break mid-morning and mid-afternoon depending on your schedule provides for your mental breather needs so you don't have a backlog to sort through when you go to bed. What you do in your brain break is up to you, but it needs to be something that doesn't require focused thought — a quick walk and a stretch, taking time out to grab a glass of water or a coffee or to have a conversation with a work colleague.

Studies have shown that taking a break with a colleague works well on several levels: it's a social opportunity to get to know your colleague a little better; and your conversation may spark a valuable insight; most importantly, though, it's time out for a rest before heading back into focused work again.

As Cal Newport, author of *Deep Work*, shares, our ability to do deep work maximises our intellectual capacity, and adhering to complete shutdown helps to separate out work thoughts from other thinking. Trying to squeeze more out of our brain in the evenings on work-related matters reduces our effectiveness the following day because it affects sleep quality. Newport believes that 'providing the conscious brain down time to rest enables your subconscious mind to take a shift sorting through your most complex professional challenges'.

How can you inject a couple more brain breaks into your day to get a better night's sleep?

 A brain break a day keeps the sleep bogeyman away.

Plan the night before

If your mind is always racing ahead, planning what's next, spending time at night in an endless loop of 'what else', taking time out at the end of the day to reflect on what went well and what you've achieved (and to congratulate yourself) helps to reduce stress. And if your typical to-do list is five A4 pages, studies have shown that writing tomorrow's to-do list using paper and pen *before* going to bed can help you fall asleep a full nine minutes sooner.

The writing part is important because it helps your brain process the information. This can also be very helpful if you've got a lot on your mind and your worries are keeping you awake. Nine minutes may not seem like much, but night after night that contributes a good amount of extra sleep time that would otherwise go to waste.

Dr Nancy Digeon found that writing in a gratitude journal for 15 minutes each night also reduced bedtime worrying and led to longer and better quality sleep. And another survey from the UK found that expressing gratitude before sleep produced more positive thoughts and led subjects to fall asleep faster and enjoy more restful sleep.

 Practising gratitude helps you sleep better.

To promote a better night's sleep, here are some basic principles to follow.

Consistency and ritual

Create your own regular bedtime routine, going to bed (recommended as between 9 and 11 pm) and getting up at a consistent time. This might sound dull, but it is the golden key to a better night's sleep. A pre-bed routine allows you to wind down to prepare for sleep. A warm bath or shower will help you fall to sleep more easily. Enjoy a herbal tea. Undertake a quiet activity such as reading or listening to some soothing music.

Get your environment right

Make sure the bedroom environment is optimised for its main purpose, with a comfortable mattress and pillows; if you use a doona, don't put a sheet between you and it as it restricts the breathability of the quilt. Keep the room dark (use blackout blinds if needed to avoid waking too early in summer), cool (between 16 and 19 degrees Celsius) and quiet. Being too hot in bed can make you restless while being too cold can keep you awake.

Light is a critical factor for sleep. The marvellous invention of the electric light bulb allowed us to extend the time spent awake, but our body has evolved to be attuned to the solar cycle.

'Lightmare', a term coined by Professor Richard G. Stevens, refers to the idea that light pollution is impacting our circadian pattern and disrupting our sleep. Circadian lighting, which exposes us to bright white light in the morning and warmer, more muted light in the evening, can help.

Switch off from your technology at least an hour before bed

The blue backlight of most screens suppresses melatonin production by your pineal gland, fooling the brain into thinking it's still daytime. So keep technology OUT of the bedroom.

This includes the TV, laptop, tablet, your mobile phone and even your digital alarm clock. If checking your mobile is the last thing you do before switching out the light and the first thing you do on waking, you're keeping your brain in a hyper-stimulated state that is not conducive to sleep.

Why not spend the time talking to your partner, undertake a meditation practice or reading a book instead? Reading can take you away from other distracting thoughts — just don't read anything too exciting!

If you have computer work you must do in the evening, try switching to a yellow backlight such as f.lux, but still allow plenty of time for your brain to relax after closing down your laptop. If you're on an iPad, though, the night shift mode has *not* been shown to reduce melatonin suppression.

What does this mean? If you're a poor sleeper, staying hooked to your technology isn't going to help your sleep pattern, but please don't stress about this, as worry will be far more effective at stopping you from sleeping than being exposed to blue light. The tech that can be helpful includes light alarms and apps that provide white noise. Our son used to complain he couldn't sleep without a fan on, because he needed the noise to drift off to sleep.

Find the time for exercise

If you've been sitting at a desk all day or in bed sick, it's harder to sleep well. A minimum of 20 minutes' exercise each day will make a big difference, as will a daily meditation session of at least 10 minutes.

Exercise is a really easy way to improve your sleep pattern. If you can't get down to the gym, look for opportunities to move around more across your day, especially if your work is predominantly sedentary in nature. Paradoxically, working out in the morning is ideal for boosting how much time you spend in deep sleep, the type of sleep associated with waking feeling refreshed, and it boosts your serotonin levels, helping you to feel calm and happy. The only caveat with exercise is to avoid it within two hours of bedtime to reduce the risk of the stress hormone cortisol produced during exercise from interfering with your sleep.

Beware of the sleep poisons

Caffeine is well known for disturbing sleep patterns because it competes with the naturally occurring brain chemical adenosine, which is produced in increasing quantities across the day, making us drowsy by day's end. Because the two molecules both fit the adenosine receptors in the brain and because caffeine has a half-life of between four and seven hours, it can block the adenosine from taking effect. While there are some fast caffeine metabolisers whose sleep patterns are less disrupted, if you're sensitive to caffeine's effect it's recommended you drink your caffeinated beverages including coffee, black tea and green tea before 2 pm.

It's common to view alcohol as a welcome way to wind down after a busy day at work but beware — it also alters how adenosine works. While you may find it easier to get to sleep after a couple of glasses of wine, that's sufficient to halve the amount of time your brain spends in REM sleep at night, disrupting memory consolidation. It's recommended that you stop drinking alcohol at least three hours before sleep. Of course, this means that you can expect to pay for a Friday night out with friends with a less than perfect night's sleep.

Worse than either alcohol or caffeine, smoking is a terrible sleep poison. Nicotine disrupts your sleep–wake cycle by altering gene expression. This can put you at increased risk of mood disorder — especially anxiety and depression — and you have two and a half times the risk of developing sleep apnoea. You can expect generally poorer sleep and greater difficulty falling asleep and maintaining sleep. So quit the smokes at least two hours before going to bed. In fact, just quit. Smoking is bad for your health and cognition. If keeping your brain in good working order as you age is important to you, this is a VERY good reason to stop now.

Try meditation

If you are a bit of a stress head or just feeling a bit down, meditation can promote a greater sense of calm and wellbeing and better sleep patterns. It quietens the mind, lowers stress hormones, and lowers your blood pressure and heart rate, making it easier to fall asleep. Mindfulness meditation focusing on the breath is easy to learn and even short sessions offer benefits. Why not sign up for a course near you to learn the skill and embed the habit?

This could be a good time to go back to the chapter on mindfulness in part II and practise the meditation exercise. In that chapter I talked about the use of sleep meditation apps. You might also want to consider yoga nidra, a yogic practice using meditation to guide you towards a deeply relaxed state while remaining inwardly alert. While research in this area is as yet limited, advocates suggest 30 minutes of yoga nigra is equivalent to two hours of deep (restorative) sleep. One study examined how the practice impacted the mental health of college professors and showed it to be helpful. Other studies found it aids blood pressure and heart rate variability and reduces emotional reactivity. If it helps, why not give it a try?

Meditation helps to reduce the weight of all that emotional baggage we so often carry around with us, making us responsive rather than reactive to our daily stresses. The total body scan, which entails conscious progressive muscular relaxation, is another great way to release tension and help your drift off to sleep more easily.

Meditation works because it strengthens the amount of time spent in deep restorative sleep and boosts melatonin production through stress reduction.

Breathe

Consciously slowing down your breathing rate influences your vagal tone to slow down your heart rate, help you relax and prepare you to fall asleep more easily.

Have a small, light carbohydrate snack before bed

This will boost serotonin levels, which assist in regulating sleep.

Take an afternoon nap

Naps are great as cognitive refreshers. If you're getting poor sleep at night, a 15- to 20-minute power nap can be a life saver. Best taken after lunch, it can boost your attention levels for several hours and top up your sleep without interfering with your nocturnal sleep pattern. Keeping the nap short keeps you in the lighter phase of sleep, which means it's easy to wake up and you won't have that horrible, groggy sense of inertia from being in a deeper phase of sleep. Best of all, you don't actually need to sleep. Just resting quietly with your eyes closed in a darkened room can provide the same benefit.

Many workplaces, especially those where a high degree of creativity and innovation is needed, now provide a nap space where tired employees can restore their attention focus and productivity. Try it — it works!

Seek help

If sleep still remains elusive and it's getting you down, it's time to seek help. Talk to your health practitioner. They may refer you for a sleep study (these now often take place in the comfort of your own home) or to a sleep specialist. With more than 80 sleep disorders to choose from, there are sure to be reasons why you're not sleeping so well. Knowing what they are and what can help is the path back to good sleep patterns.

Cognitive behavioural therapy (CBT-i) has an excellent track record for helping those with various forms of chronic insomnia — difficulty falling or maintaining sleep or waking too early.

Obstructive sleep apnoea is a dangerous sleep disorder in which you stop breathing multiple times during the night, reducing the oxygen supply to your brain. If you are a heavy snorer (your partner will tell you!) or they've noticed you stop breathing during sleep (which is quite alarming to observe) and you're chronically tired during the day please, see your doctor. There are a number of management strategies to help including CPAP, weight reduction if obesity is a factor, and other appliances.

Poor sleep is frequently a signal that something else in your life is wrong so ask your health practitioner for a full assessment to get to the root of the problem and work out the most effective treatment plan.

 Poor sleep is often an indicator that something else is not right in your life.

Your prescription for a better night's sleep

- Make getting enough sleep non-negotiable.

- Consistency, consistency, consistency. Make the timing of your sleeping hours a consistent habit.

- Prepare for a great night's sleep with a wind-down routine: put away all your toys, have a nice warm bath and put on your 'jammies' before having your bedtime story.

- Manage any worries by using a pre-sleep meditation, keeping a gratitude journal or writing down your plans for tomorrow.

- Keep your sleep cave cool, dark and comfy, and restrict it for sleep and sex.

- Getting enough sleep means you'll get more out of every day, with the energy and alertness to keep you focused and on track, and a positive mood to keep you feeling happy and ready to deal with the day's events with greater curiosity and calm.

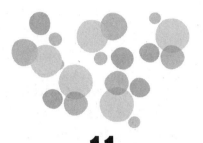

11
Food to boost your mood

There was an Old Man from Putney
Whose food was roast spiders and chutney
Which he took with his tea,
In sight of the sea
That romantic Old Man from Putney.
Edward Lear

You know how it goes. You're busy, got stuff to do and there's no time to think about what to eat, let alone plan what's for dinner. When it's presented you eat it, or you grab something on the go because there's always the next meeting scheduled, flight to catch or client to entertain.

But you've got no energy. You're iron deficient, feel like crap and are gaining weight. What's going on?

Whether you're a CEO in New York, a GM in Dubai, a small business owner in Sydney or a busy professional in Japan, we all need the right fuel to nourish our bodies and provide the building blocks for maintenance and repair so we can think clearly and maintain a positive mood.

There's just one problem.

 The way we live, work and interact with the world has changed, and so has the food we eat.

It's easy to point the finger of blame for our rising levels of anxiety and depression on our super-stressful, sleep-deprived and hectic lifestyle, but then we're missing something else, something so basic to human health and wellbeing we often forget to even consider it.

Our food.

Who do you take your dietary advice from? Because it seems every man, woman and dog has an opinion on what's best to eat and if you don't agree, look out! With the surfeit of conflicting information, celebrity cookbooks and fad diets doing the rounds, it can be more than a tad confusing to decide who to believe any more. Should you follow Paleo Pete, Keto Kitty or Viktor Vegan?

What's important is to understand that food choices matter. What you put in your mouth has the potential to impact your physical and mental wellbeing, emotions, state of mind and thinking skills. The existing data is compelling but remains incomplete, because our understanding relating to the *microbiome* remains very much in its infancy. It's time to tune in to what the nutritionists and food scientists have discovered in order to build a sound basis for our beliefs.

What we've learned from the Blue Zones

When we speak of the Blue Zones we are referring to a number of widely dispersed regions scattered around the world where the inhabitants have been found to live exceptionally long, healthy and active lives. One factor common to all these communities is a shared belief in the importance of eating fresh, locally sourced food and using food as a means to stay socially connected.

With diet such an important contributor to our overall health and wellbeing, if you are the driver of the shopping trolley or in charge of the online shopping order, remember your choices will impact your own and your family's health today and for the years to come.

 Your food choices determine your health and mental wellbeing.

The brainy facts about food and mental health

Even a couple of years ago, the idea of using food to help manage mental mood disorders and maintain mental wellbeing would have been laughed out of court. But the new field of nutritional psychiatry is now leading the way.

Nutritional researcher Felice Jacka and her team at Deakin University's Mood and Food Centre led the SMILES Trial, hailed as an important first step in demonstrating the role of food on mood. This study sought to answer the question of whether dietary intervention (that is, improving diet) could be useful as an adjunct treatment strategy for depression, and the results indicated a big fat yes.

In the trial, 67 subjects with clinically diagnosed moderate to severe depression were enrolled to receive either dietary or social support. Fifty-five of the group were currently using medication and/or psychotherapy. Over a 12-week period the group on dietary support were put on the Modified Mediterranean Diet, which focuses on 12 key food groups: whole grains, vegetables, fruit, legumes, low-fat and unsweetened dairy foods, raw and unsalted nuts, fish, lean red meat, chicken, eggs and olive oil. Their intake of extras — sweets, refined cereals, fried food, fast foods, processed meats and sugary drinks — was reduced.

The primary outcome? A significant reduction in symptoms of depression in the dietary support group.

While no one is proposing that diet alone is the solution to mood disorders such as depression, it's clear our diet has a role to play, and if it means feeling less depressed, recovering more quickly or needing lower doses of anti-depressants, that has to be a big plus.

Have you ever wondered what our current SAD (Standard American/Australian Diet) is doing to us? With one in five adults at risk of developing a mental health disorder in any 12 months, think of the gains to be made in lowering that potential risk and reducing the impact of mental mood disorders by choosing to pay closer attention to our diet.

The link between fast food and depression is real and given the dose-response relationship the more fast food we eat, especially with added refined sugar, the higher the risk of developing depression.

With depression known to have the same impact on our mortality as smoking, how can you ensure you are eating well for your mental health?

Optimal nutrition is about balance and meeting our nutritional needs at every age by eating as wide a range of healthy, unprocessed foods as possible. Until more data from random controlled trials become available nutritionists recommend a predominantly plant-based diet that is anti-inflammatory and high in vitamins, fibre and unsaturated fat. Besides the Mediterranean diet, other healthy diets include the Nordic, Japanese, MIND and DASH diets. It's time to move away from the traditional Western meat-and-two-veg paradigm towards adopting a plant-based focus with a side of protein, whether derived from animal products or from foods such as legumes and nuts.

What one small change can you make to your diet to reduce the risk of poorer mental wellbeing?

Cutting down on processed foods, takeaways and soft drinks would be a great start.

Introducing small changes to your diet is less stressful and more sustainable. Thinking of it as an invitation to change rather than a command also helps. Taste buds can be re-educated with repeated exposure to a new food.

Planning is key in the brave new world of healthy nutrition. Check out the location of your nearest farmers market and get organised. Cooking in bulk and freezing portions is a huge time saver for those busy nights when the alternative would be takeaway.

Offer lots of new tastes and snack foods to develop new favourites and healthy options.

Be prepared. If Wednesday and Thursday nights at work often run late, have some healthy alternatives at the ready, so when the call goes out for 'Let's get pizza!' you've got a healthier alternative waiting.

Food is a terrific connector

Food is commonly shared. Whether we're celebrating a birthday, a significant milestone or any other special event we like to base the occasion on the social context of food:

- 'Come to dinner' is a way we catch up with friends and family.

- A working lunch with your colleagues facilitates the sharing of ideas while ensuring you don't end up working all afternoon on an empty stomach.

- My personal favourite? Breakfast out, where you get to enjoy healthy food options and a lazy cup of coffee, and don't have to worry about the washing up. Bliss!

Have you noticed how we eat differently in the company of others? Robin Dunbar from the University of Oxford found the more often people eat together, the more likely they are to have a wider social network that provides social and emotional support, to feel happy and to report being satisfied with their lives.

But busy and hectic lives can make this hard. In the UK one-third of evening meals are eaten alone, and the average person eats 10 of their 21 meals in isolation. Planning and prepping for one is a vastly different prospect from preparing a meal for four or six. The option of grabbing a takeaway tends to be more appealing if you're eating alone.

Obstacles in our way

There are many reasons why we don't always opt for the healthier food choice, including:

- **personal preference**. How fussy are you?

- **availability**. It's after hours and your choice is between the snack bar vending machine and the fast-food outlet that's open 24/7

- **lack of culinary skills.** My dad never cooked anything more than baked beans on toast his entire life. He had no interest in learning to cook, choosing to rely on Mum's ability and dietetics training to provide him with what he liked

- eating for comfort or out of boredom, rather than hunger.

Identifying what drives you to eat beyond hunger is the first step towards finding a way to make healthier choices.

Why our emotions drive us to eat

In our high-stress environments, emotional eating is very common, especially on those days when nothing's gone right and we're desperately seeking solace in food, alcohol or other reward. The problem here is we're not satisfied with just one biscuit out of the packet; we want to consume the whole thing, along with two litres of ice cream and the family-sized bar of chocolate we've had hidden at the back of the pantry.

You might gain some short-term emotional relief from this self-indulgence, but in the longer term gorging on those high-fat, high-sugar foods actually makes you feel worse. Consuming excessive amounts of sugar triggsers inflammation and that's bad for body and brain.

It's recommended that you restrict your refined sugar intake to 25 grams (six teaspoons) a day. The average Australian consumes around 68 grams.

In a longitudinal prospective study of more than 10 300 male and female civil servants, researchers examined the impact of sugar consumption on mood disorder. They found that men who consumed the most sugar over the long term had a 23 per cent increased risk of developing a mood disorder over time. Other research also linked excess refined sugar consumption (and artificial sweeteners) to higher levels of neuroinflammation leading to brain disease and memory problems.

If stress is your dietary downfall, what measures can you put in place that you have found effective in allowing you to enjoy a small treat without lapsing into a binge?

Emotional eating is a maladaptive response to dealing with stress.

.The two most commonly cited reasons for why we don't always make the healthiest food choices are, unsurprisingly, money and time.

Healthy food is expensive

Cost is one of the most common reasons given by my patients for not making healthier food choices. But need this be true?

Felice Jacka's research included comparing the costs of the group's normal (generally unhealthy) diet with the Modified Mediterranean Diet, and guess what — the healthier version was also the cheapest.

Lack of time

If working long hours, always running late and lacking time to get to the shops means all your fridge has to offer is an out-of-date tub of yoghurt and half a tin of dog meat for Fido, it's going to be hard to find the inspiration, energy or interest in 'plating up' your latest MasterChef special.

We all have a choice to make. What will yours be?

Your microbiome and you

There's been a lot in the news about our gut microbiome lately. Everyone wants to know more about the trillions of bacteria and viruses that inhabit our gut and contribute to our health and well-being. Our interest has been piqued by the new science and some of the discoveries have challenged long-held beliefs and provided fresh insights into the causes of some diseases.

If you still think you use your brain to make your dietary choices, think again, because that craving you've got for mac 'n cheese or a chocolate muffin with apple and raspberries is being directed by something other than you.

Let me introduce you to your microbiome.

Your microbiome comprises the 100 trillion bacteria, viruses, parasites and fungi that cover our body and inhabit our gut. We've known of its existence for a long time, but it's only relatively recently that it has begun giving up some of its secrets, enhancing our understanding of different disease processes that affect the human body and leading to potential novel approaches to their treatment and management. This new understanding is revealing how making better food choices can tip the balance towards better general health, including better brain health and mental wellbeing.

While the thought of having all these microbes living inside us might be alarming, we can draw comfort from the knowledge that they've been our constant companions throughout our evolutionary history. Most of them contribute to our wellbeing, but as in any good story, there are always a couple of dastardly villains that seek to cause us harm, as you may remember from the last time you ate a dodgy chicken curry.

All these microbes help us digest our food, produce vitamins B and K, fight inflammation through the production of immune molecules and create neurotransmitters identical to the ones produced by the brain including serotonin, which helps to regulate emotion. Ninety per cent of our serotonin is produced in the gut, not the brain.

Your gut microbes are special because they behave as independent janitors of your gut health, communicating with and directing your gut and brain via the bi-directional gut–brain axis, and the healthiest microbiome is the one that's the most diverse, obtained through eating a wide variety of different foods. Cutting out entire food groups is never a good way to achieve a balanced diet.

The best diet is the one that provides the greatest variety of nutrients.

Cultivating a healthy microbiome

Your microbiome is in constant flux, meaning the balance of different bacteria changes with virtually every meal. Think of it as though you're eating for two — yourself and your microbiome. Keeping your microbiome healthy moves you towards better health. This means including lots of lovely fibre (or what my dad liked to call 'roughage') in your diet. You may not be able to digest all those fibrous foods, but your gut microbes love them. A three-hat Michelin meal for your gut microbes would include lots of *prebiotics*, such as garlic, onions, leeks, asparagus, green bananas (high in resistant starch), oats, barley, apples, flaxseed, cocoa, wheat bran and seaweed.

Probiotics are those foods full of healthy microbes that help to maintain the balance of the good and bad microbes in your gut. All the fermented foods often helpfully labelled as containing live cultures feature here, including yoghurt, kefir, kimchi, kombucha, sauerkraut, tempeh, natto, miso, traditional buttermilk, Gouda, mozzarella, cheddar and cottage cheese, and pickled gherkins (fermented in brine not vinegar).

Look to include predominantly plant-based whole foods, so lots of vegetables, fruits (especially berries), lean protein (you don't have to be vegetarian or vegan), seeds and nuts, some dairy (yoghurt and some cheeses), legumes, whole grains and olive oil.

Easy as, except this doesn't reflect the typical Western diet, which is high in the sugar, fat and salt found in processed foods. The best first step is to look for ways to cut the crap from your diet. Start by replacing one takeaway meal with a home-cooked alternative or at least one of the freshly prepared meals now being offered by some supermarkets for the time poor or poor cooks.

You can change your microbiome by changing what you eat.

Changing your food preferences

Choosing to make small, positive, incremental changes to your diet will change your food preferences. Yes, you can start to develop a taste for Brussels sprouts (they are delicious roasted or thinly sliced in a salad) and nudge yourself towards greater health.

The key is to set the bar low and progress slowly. Radicalising your diet overnight is a sure-fire recipe for failure because you've spent a lifetime evolving habits and preferences around what you eat. It's unrealistic to implement big changes on Sunday and expect them to last beyond Tuesday.

It's time to be honest about the quality of your current diet. If you're already doing well, bravo, keep up the great work. If you're eating takeaway every night and the only green item on your plate is the mould from leaving it out unwashed overnight, there may be room for improvement. It helps to know that even the fussiest eaters can make a positive change.

Our dietary habits are complex though sometimes a bit limited. My little brother survived for most of his early childhood on fried eggs, chips and porridge. Fortunately, Mum didn't believe in buying snack foods so at least crisps, sweets and soft drink were off the menu. Happily, as he matured, his culinary tastes broadened to include meat, vegetables and fruit, though he'll run a mile if you wave so much as a fish finger in his direction. He doesn't do fish or any form of seafood, though he is an absolute fiend for cheese. Remember to hide it if he ever comes around to your house for a meal.

If you're not especially interested in food and yes, I have met those who see food as a bore and would happily swallow a food capsule like David Bowie's Major Tom, you could be at risk of missing out on all the essential nutrients required for good health. Fad diets that restrict particular foods or even entire food groups are not consistent with optimal eating, even when endorsed by a celebrity. Being famous, strange to tell, doesn't necessarily qualify them as having any scientific understanding of nutrition.

Shifting food preferences to improve the health of your microbiome or change its composition isn't easy. In cases of severe bowel disease such as ulcerative colitis and Crohn's disease, faecal transplants (yes, we're talking poo here) have enjoyed significant success in repopulating diseased guts with healthy bacteria from donors.

There are no short cuts to a healthy diet

I'm often asked whether it's a good idea to take dietary supplements. The short answer is no, unless you have been diagnosed with a specific nutritional deficiency, in which case talk to your health practitioner about which supplement to take and for how long.

If you know your diet could be better, swallowing a handful of expensive vitamins and minerals isn't the solution. As Professor Tom Sanders from King's College London says, 'You can't turn a bad diet into a good diet with a handful of pills'.

Nutritional supplements are a $50 billion industry and of course the manufacturers want you to consume as many of their products as they can persuade you to buy. And their marketing is clearly working when you consider that 75 per cent of Americans, 70 per cent of Australians and 34 per cent of Britons use dietary supplements regularly.

The better and cheaper option is to seek ways to improve your diet and gain some real benefit, rather than relying on supplements that don't change dietary preferences or eating habits.

As for your mental health, a report published in 2019 by the Global Council on Brain Health, an independent collaboration between scientists, health professionals, scholars and policy experts from around the world, indicated that for the small number of dietary supplements that have been well researched, there are *no demonstrable benefits to brain health* in people with normal nutrient levels. They advise: 'Save your money, honey! The GCBH does not recommend ANY dietary supplement for brain health'.

Their recommendations include the following:

1. Get your nutrients for better brain health from your diet.

2. Don't take any supplements before consulting your health care provider.

3. Check on doses, as some vitamins and minerals taken in large doses can be harmful to health.

4. There is insufficient evidence that supplements (beyond treating known Vitamin B12, folate or Vitamin D deficiency) are helpful.

5. Verify the quality and purity of ingredients as this can be highly variable.

6. Save your money; think before you buy.

7. Read the labels very carefully.

8. Check for warnings and cautions related to your particular health conditions.

There are a couple of aspects of our daily diet I frequently get asked about. So at the risk of being accused of cherry picking certain topics let's look at the role of coffee, wine, chocolate and Brussels sprouts.

Okay, I'm not actually including anything on Brussels, other than simply to say they are divine roasted and well worth a try if you've only ever known the overcooked soggy variety that's never worthy of a place on your dinner plate.

Please tell me coffee is still okay

If the thought of having to forgo your morning cuppa or favourite barista coffee is giving you conniptions, fear not, I have good news to share.

There are a lot of positives provided by our favourite caffeinated beverage, as long as we don't overdo it. How much is too much? Recent findings suggest that up to five cups of average-strength coffee is fine, depending on your individual constitution. You know how much caffeine your system tolerates, so stick with that. The five cups is the upper recommended limit. Beyond that, your relative risk of heart disease starts to climb (just saying).

Now you've stopped palpitating (or was that the caffeine?), here are some of the benefits:

⚜ It enhances our level of alertness.

⚜ It makes us more social if we drink a cup before a meeting (perhaps not if we have seven or eight meetings back to back though).

⚜ It helps us to remember learnt information (great if you're studying for exams).

⚜ It is considered a neuroprotective against dementia.

⚜ It reduces your overall risk of dying by 10 to 15 per cent compared with non–coffee drinkers, which is put down to its anti-inflammatory effect and improved use of insulin by the body.

It's a fantastic social connector. Whether for a business meeting, a casual catch-up or just something nice to do, we love going to our local café to meet and spend time with other people. Originating with the introduction of the first coffee houses in London in the mid to late 1600s, coffee drinking and social interaction have a long and happy history. Yes, coffee is appropriate to include in a healthy diet.

Glad to have put a smile on your face.

And wine?

I was waiting for that question.

The goalposts for what constitutes healthy drinking have shifted significantly and while I may be accused of being the Fun Police, the truth is that while drinking some alcohol may be better for our overall health than being teetotal, the benefits of enjoying a superb Chardonnay or Shiraz, beyond the social aspects, the pleasure of it and as a means to relax and unwind, are small and the previously held belief that red wine is good for our heart is wishful thinking.

Current Australian recommendations are as follows:

- Enjoy one standard drink (10 g alcohol) in any given 24 hours, or two at the most. Check the alcohol content of the bottle of wine you are drinking to see how many standard drinks it contains.

- Aim to keep to below 10 standard drinks a week, and include several alcohol-free days. Four or more drinks on a single occasion is considered unsafe drinking.

- Do not provide the under-18s with alcohol. Their brains are still developing and they can't process alcohol as effectively as adults.

The recommended limits are now the same for men and women, though the guidelines vary from country to country:

- in the UK, 100 g (six glasses) of wine a week

- in Europe, 150 g per week

- in the US, 196 g for men and 98 g for women.

The lack of consensus is troubling but the underlying message is the same:

 There is no safe limit for alcohol.

Is chocolate on the safe list?

It's okay, you can breathe again because, yes, a little bit of chocolate, especially dark chocolate that contains 75 per cent or higher cocoa solids, is actually good for us. Hurrah!

It's the cacao that provides the benefits of all those lovely polyphenols that in high concentrations aid our cognition, memory and mood.

If you're wondering what's the difference between cacao and cocoa, cacao is made by cold pressing unroasted cacao beans while cocoa powder is obtained by roasting raw cacao. To add to the confusion, labelling on food products is frequently inconsistent. Cacao has higher nutritional value, but consuming standard dark chocolate in moderation (because it is still a calorie-dense, high-fat food) is fine.

Eating chocolate is a great source of pleasure because it is a source of andapamide, the neurotransmitter that binds to cannabinoid receptors in the brain, inducing a sense of happiness and wellbeing, and of course doing something we enjoy also increases the release of dopamine.

Little wonder a review of eight studies examining the impact of chocolate on mood showed a positive effect on lowering depression and anxiety and elevating a sense of calm.

A metanalysis in 2012 found eating chocolate is associated with:

⊹ lower blood pressure

⊹ reduced insulin resistance

- improved blood vessel function
- improved cholesterol ratios – lower LGL cholesterol and higher HDH
- lower triglyceride leve0ls
- elevated mood (the magnesium in chocolate is believed to lower cortisol and improve mood, memory, focus and sleep)
- sharper memory (from the caffeine effect)
- positive effect on the microbiome.

I think that's enough proof. Case closed.

Just remember we're talking about a couple of small squares of top-quality chocolate, not the entire family bar of 'Fruit and Nut'.

Eating well for your future

Have you noticed how when you've been eating well you have more energy, feel more vital and enjoy a more positive state of mind? One of the most common comments I hear from clients who have made the change to eating a predominantly whole foods diet is just how much more energised they feel on waking up in the morning, how they're set up to enjoy a great day.

By contrast, food that is calorie dense and nutritionally poor puts us at greater risk of weight gain and chronic conditions such as type 2 diabetes, heart disease and depression. Processed food, baked goods, pastries and pies are linked to the excessive consumption of trans fats (the by-products of hydrogenised oils), which increases your risk of heart disease, stroke and type 2 diabetes with higher levels of LDL and lower levels of HDL cholesterol. Worse still, they have been linked to memory problems in men.

It's time to plan ahead and choose to include those food items in the shopping trolley to boost your mood, general health and social connection. If your diet is lacking, start to cut out the rubbish and follow author Michael Pollan's recommendation to 'eat real food, not too much, mostly plants'.

Your prescription for healthier eating

- Make the decision to eat more healthily.

- Give yourself permission to do so.

- Tell someone – your partner, a friend or colleague – what you're doing so they can help keep you accountable.

- Run a reality check for a typical day; be honest – this is for your benefit. How well do you eat on a normal day? If there's room for improvement, perhaps look for ways to reduce your intake of processed foods or foods high in added refined sugar, salt or saturated fat.

- Create a plan, with a start date and a reward for successful completion of the task at the end of the week (maybe not a donut).

- Choose one thing to make a point of difference:

  - Swap soft drink for water (tap, filtered or carbonated, but not flavoured or vitamin enhanced).

  - Swap a daytime treat for a healthy, yummy alternative. Hummus and vegetable sticks, a piece of fruit or small handful of nuts.

  - Add an extra green vegetable to your evening meal.

  - Take a proper lunchbreak away from your desk. 'Al desko' is mindless eating.

  - Opt for a meatless meal once a week and go for legumes (such as chickpeas or lentils) to add more fibre to your diet.

- Put the money saved from not getting a takeaway towards something you'd really like.

- Be mindful of your food when preparing, cooking, tasting and eating it.

- Get adventurous. Never eaten couscous or made chocolate and avocado tart? Surprise yourself and your tastebuds by trying out new foods and flavour combinations.

- Keep it simple. Sometimes it's the simplest of dishes that provide the greatest delight, such as *Insalata caprese*, combining sliced fresh tomatoes (that haven't been refrigerated and lost their flavour), buffalo mozzarella, a little olive oil and balsamic vinegar, black pepper and a couple of fresh basil leaves. *Delizioso!*

- Enjoy your special occasional treats without guilt and savour every last morsel.

- Choose to change your relationship with food to one that is supportive, enjoyable and social.

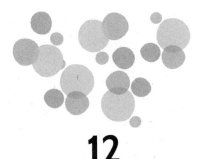

12

Exercise
as medicine

*The single most important daytime activity for better health,
smarter thinking and greater happiness is to stay on your feet
and keep moving.*
J.B.

I have a confession to make. As a child I hated sport.

Short-sighted, knock-kneed, asthmatic and with a poor sense
of visuospatial awareness I was never the PE teacher's darling.
In short, I was ignored. We both knew I was never going to
play sport for the school. I specialised in trying to make myself
invisible, hiding behind the sports bags in the locker room to
avoid the ignominy of being the last person chosen to join a team
or running out of breath and turning blue on the hockey pitch.
Unfortunately, my cunning plan never worked.

While I admired the prowess of those who made delivering
the tennis ball accurately to the other end of the court look so

easy (my hits had an uncanny knack of ending up on the court next door), I was far happier as a cheerleader than a participant.

We weren't taught about the benefits of exercise at medical school, which suited me fine as my focus was on trying to pass all the exams.

It wasn't until my Gap Year that I came to understand my perspective towards exercise was somewhat narrow. That was when we got our first dog, and he needed his daily walk, and since I was the one at home, naturally it fell to me to provide it. Starting with short walks around the block, Homer and I began to explore the suburb we had lived in for a couple of decades but hardly knew because I'd always been elsewhere. I discovered pockets of green, paths and small ovals between the houses and protected bushland I never knew existed. I started to enjoy our daily forays, which became longer and were taken at a brisker pace. Soon I came to realise not only that I looked forward to our walks, but that they were helping me to feel better too. My walks were making me happier.

Now exercise is a daily feature of my life. The walks have continued—Homer and I would be equally bereft if they stopped—but I have also discovered the pleasures of other physical activities, notably swimming, cycling and Pilates. Now I go a little stir-crazy if I don't get out and move regularly. Today exercise is one of the daily strategies I use to manage my stress and think better. Some of my best ideas have come to me while walking along the beach or following that black line in the swimming pool.

 Exercise is the single most effective method to live, think and age well.

The power of exercise

Exercise keeps us fitter, healthier, thinking better and mentally well. Think of it as medicine to alleviate symptoms of stress, anxiety and depression, protect your brain from the ageing process and help you stay cognitively sharp, make smarter decisions and manage your emotions more effectively.

With so much going for exercise, surely we should be bottling it up and drinking it as the elixir of life?

Except we aren't.

Well, some are. As far as exercise goes, you can classify people into three general groups:

1. those who have always loved it, even when it hurts, and can't imagine life without it

2. those who don't, because all that hot sweaty stuff just seems like too much hard work and effort and they'd much rather watch the rugby, cricket or tennis on the telly than take part in it themselves

3. the 'shouldas', who bear the burden of good intentions, and understand the benefits, but somehow never quite get down to the gym, get the bike out of the garage or know where those trainers are hiding.

Which category do you fit into? Is exercise and being physically active a joy or is the thought of wearing Lycra® enough to bring you out in a rash? If you're a *shoulda, coulda* or *woulda* wondering how the heck to get started, or are seeking the motivation and inspiration to start back up again after falling off the exercise wagon when life or work took over, this chapter is for you.

Roughly 44 per cent of Australians are sufficiently physically active. They have made exercise part of who they are and what they do. They get up in the morning and scoot off to the gym or cycle 50 kilometres before breakfast or row on the river for 40 minutes, and still get to work on time. Fortunately, many employers supply showers and change facilities to reduce the incidence of stale sweat and smelly socks in the workplace.

But according to the Australian Health Survey, 20 per cent of adult Australians fail to undertake *any* regular physical exercise and more than 30 per cent don't achieve the recommended minimum of 150 minutes per week.

Across the Pacific, Americans fare even worse. *Mayo Clinic Proceedings* reports that less than 3 per cent of Americans meet the basic qualifications for a healthy lifestyle (oops, I think that reads 'room for improvement') and only 20 per cent meet exercise guidelines.

Globally, one in four adults and three in four adolescents (aged 11–17) fail to meet the minimum recommendation for exercise.

It's not that we don't know how important exercise is to our health and wellbeing; it's about knowing how to overcome the three major obstacles of:

* time
* fatigue
* not having a form of exercise you think you would enjoy.

If only I had more time

Actually, you have all the time you need. If prioritising your own self-care is proving tricky, is it time to give yourself permission to make the time available? What can you shift, defer or delete to create the time required?

I'm too tired

This is a common problem. The question to ask is what's causing you to be so darn tired in the first place and how can you start fixing that? Are you working too many hours, doing too much for everyone else or not getting enough sleep?

The paradox is that undertaking even a small amount of regular exercise is energising. So if you're home late and thinking you've already missed the first half of your yoga session so you won't bother going, what if you went anyway and got half a class done, or rescheduled for another time so as to not miss out?

There's nothing about exercise I enjoy

Call it something else. If it's the E word you find distressing, how does dance sound? Loathe the gym? How about kicking a ball around with the kids or playing some backyard cricket (and not just at Christmas)? Undertaking a physical activity in company shifts the focus from exercise to having fun.

Remember the new exercise prescription:

 Move more, sit less.

It's not that we don't know how good exercise is for us. The problems lie elsewhere:

1. How do we incorporate sufficient exercise into our ridiculously busy lives without it feeling a burden or a chore, making it something that just happens, without hassle, something we look forward to?

2. How can we come to love exercise when it's something we studiously try to avoid or actively dislike? Hint: This is about *why* exercise is so important and *how* a little reframing can make all the difference.

Still looking for inspiration? Let's take a look at why exercise is so important.

The brainy benefits of exercise

If you've ever left your car sitting in the garage for too long without using it, the risk is the battery will have gone flat or the engine has developed problems. In just the same way you need to keep your body moving to keep your health and wellbeing in tip-top condition.

Exercise and mental wellbeing

You may have noticed how when you've got a lot on your mind going for a walk or a jog helps to clarify your thoughts. You come back feeling energised and in a better mood. And because the effect results from that boost in blood flow and release of neurochemicals, exercising earlier in the day is ideal.

Research has shown that regular exercisers enjoy better mental wellbeing, with an average of 18 fewer days of feeling bad compared with the less physically active.

In his book *Spark!*, John Ratey identified the cognitive and emotional benefits of exercising at the beginning of the day. But if that thought sends you into a complete tailspin because of all the other activities that consume your mornings, *any* time (except within two or three hours of bedtime) is good.

A number of studies have confirmed that supervised aerobic exercise has an antidepressant effect through boosting the release of the powerful mood-enhancing hormones dopamine, serotonin and endorphins. No wonder a little bit of exercise makes us feel good.

Exercise for longevity

Taking a brisk 25-minute walk every day (taking the dog is optional but enjoyable for both) can add between three and seven years to your life by reducing the risk of depression and potentially warding off cognitive decline. Now there's a bonus.

Exercise for smarter thinking and better memory

Research from the University of British Columbia has shown how regular aerobic exercise, the sort that makes you huff and puff, increases the size of the hippocampus, the part of the brain used for learning and verbal memory. It's also the first part of the brain affected by Alzheimer's, which is why exercise is so critical to your future brain health.

Building extra brain power can be achieved by undertaking regular, moderate-intensity exercise such as a brisk one-hour walk twice a week for six to 12 months. Research by neurologist Scott McGinnis at Brigham and Women's Hospital found that this moderate aerobic exercise led to an increase in volume of the prefrontal cortex and medial temporal cortex, the brain areas involved in controlling thinking and memory.

The effect of exercise is felt fast. A single session is enough to elevate your attentional skills and focus for two hours as well as increase your reaction time. If you're feeling a little sluggish and it's only 9.30 in the morning, rather than hanging out for yet another coffee, why not get out for a quick walk or jog around the block and start to get fitter, faster and happier too. Your brain will thank you for it.

Exercise and happiness

Science tells us exercise significantly boosts our happiness and reduces symptoms of anxiety, depression and stress. One large international study found that an hour of exercise a week reduced the risk of future depression by 15 per cent, with the protective effect rising to 22 per cent if the recommended 150 minutes per week was reached. Not a bad ROI for avoiding a debilitating and potentially lethal illness.

Elsewhere American researchers found exercising regularly for 30 to 60 minutes is the ideal to reduce the number of mental health days taken, especially when participating in team sports, going to the gym, aerobics and cycling.

In this study researchers from Yale and Oxford asked 1.2 million Americans the question, 'How many times have you felt mentally unwell in the last thirty days due to stress, depression or emotional worries?' They found that being more physically active equated to feeling as good as the group who weren't active but earned $25 000 more, indicating the strength of the happiness-boosting effect of exercise.

The positive benefits are quickly achieved. Just 20 minutes of exercise have been shown to boost your mood for up to 12 hours, according to researchers from the University of Vermont. If you're in a bit of a funk, getting out for that 20 minutes can make a huge difference to the rest of your day. You'll get a better result from a sustained 20 to 30 minutes rather than several shorter exercise breaks.

If life has lost some of its sparkle, regular exercise can help you extract more pleasure from your days, even when nothing else has changed.

The protective effect of exercise comes from being active whatever your age; it's never too late to start and gain the benefits.

If you're studying hard for exams, reducing stress through exercise is a great way to maintain a clear head and achieve better learning, and you'll be feeling stronger and fitter too.

 ## It's time to stand up for greater mental wellbeing.

In summary, exercise:

- promotes neuroplasticity and neurogenesis, keeping your brain working well

- reduces brain shrinkage, preserving your smarts and reducing your risk of dementia

- enhances cognitive function, priming the brain to learn, stay focused, lay down new memory, instil new habits and create new ideas

- is energising, increasing muscle strength and endurance

- improves your physical health, lowering your risk of heart disease, stroke and type 2 diabetes

- elevates the production of your feel-good hormones, causing you to feel happier

- helps to burn off the stress hormone cortisol
- protects against the development and relapse of mood disorders such as anxiety and depression
- helps you to keep your emotions and perspective in check
- promotes better sleep patterns
- assists in recall of information when needed
- helps you to maintain a healthy weight.

How much exercise do you need?

The recommendation is 150 minutes of moderate-intensity or 75 minutes of intense aerobic exercise per week spread out as best suits you, *plus* a couple of sessions of weight training (resistance exercises) a week.

Why not look to start with three to five sessions of 30 to 60 minutes and build from there, gradually increasing the intensity and duration of your workout?

How do you structure your exercise routine?

During the week I aim to walk every day for 30 to 40 minutes, while on the weekends, with the luxury of more time available, there's nothing I enjoy more than getting out for a longer hike in the bush or walk along the beach. I include two to three 50-minute combined cardio-Pilates classes each week, and also aim to squeeze in a swim or cycle ride.

A cautionary note: As with many things there is an upper limit of what is safe. It's been found that overexercising — more than 23 sessions in a month or working out for longer than three hours a day — is associated with worse mental health!

10 000 steps?

If you've been listening to the public health messages 'Find thirty!' or '10,000 steps a day', you might be disappointed to discover you've been duped. There's nothing magical or mysterious about 30 minutes' exercise or 10 000 steps. It was a clever marketing ploy to sell new-fangled pedometers at the 1964 Tokyo Olympics which first introduced the nice round number of *Manpo-kei* (10 000 steps) as a minimum to aim for to fight the risk of high blood pressure, type 2 diabetes and stroke.

When 10 000 steps came to be adopted as the new walking mantra around the world, questions began to be asked. Did the number have any scientific basis? The Department of Movement and Sports Sciences at Ghent University in Belgium in conjunction with its counterpart at the University of Queensland showed that adhering to the 10 000 steps goal is of value for boosting health and wellbeing, but only if it is maintained.

Rather than any arbitrary number of steps, it is the consistency of regular activity that matters. Making walking part of your everyday routine will guarantee you the improved health benefits of being more active, whether you walk 6000 steps or more.

For your fitness tracker to be more useful than just as a social indicator of your potential interest in staying physically fit, let's examine how measuring your daily activity can be a useful metric and guide for monitoring your level of physical activity. If the number is disappointingly low (*Surely I've been more active than that!*), it's a useful reality check.

It's been shown that the benefit of upping your activity is greatest when starting from the lower end of the physical activity scale. The person who currently does very little exercise will benefit most from achieving 2000 to 4000 steps a day, but almost all of us can benefit from doing a little bit more.

Cheating is not useful. Waving your arms about to raise the score doesn't count. If you're a big gesticulator, sorry but your conversation with friends doesn't actually count as part of your exercise regime.

Consistent daily activity is key.

Does it matter what type of exercise I do? In a word, no. What matters is finding something you like doing and making it a regular habit. As far as your brain is concerned, *all* physical activity counts. If triathlons are your thing, fantastic, but otherwise look to include a variety of different activities to help prevent boredom.

For more information on different forms of exercise, head to the resource page link on my website, www.drjennybrockis. com/resources

 Exercise is the single most important thing you can do for your health and wellbeing.

Sitting: the new smoking

With so much going for being physically active, the paradox is that for a number of reasons we have become increasingly sedentary. This comes at a terrible cost: for 2013 this was estimated at INT$54 billion in direct costs (2013) plus $14 billion in indirect costs.

According to a report in *The Lancet*, physical inactivity is the fourth leading risk factor for death in the world,

The thing to remember is that a single session of exercise cannot make up for the negative effects of sitting on our bottom all day. Seeking out opportunities to move more and sit less is the way to go.

How long do you think you sit for each day? This should include the time spent eating, commuting, at work and relaxing. Many of us spend more time sitting on our backside than we do lying in our beds. The average person sits for 62 per cent of their day.

 Our sedentary lifestyle is killing us.

Sorry to be blunt. But the solution is simple. Make the choice to stand up and move around more across your day. Note to the exercise-phobe and activity intolerant: This is not about Activewear© or Spanx© undergarments, or training for the next Olympics, merely about getting up out of your chair and moving, because:

We think better on our feet

Anti-sedentary campaigns now encourage us to think before we sit. The 2015 consensus statement commissioned and released by Public Health England and the Active Working Community Interest Company aimed to provide guidance for office workers to combat the problems of sedentary work by encouraging individuals to move towards two hours a day of standing and light activity (walking), progressing to four hours a day.

The Get Britain Standing organisation is spreading the word to help us make the better choice by providing evidence that sitting for eight hours a day:

- raises your risk of heart disease, cancer and diabetes by 40 per cent
- increases your risk of a fatal heart attack by 64 per cent
- slows your rate of metabolism dramatically.

Tips to reduce your sitting time

- Stand while enjoying a coffee break or eating your lunch.
- Get out for a stroll, run or jog during your lunchbreak.

- Stand when making or taking a phone call.

- Choose to stand on the bus, train or ferry on your commute.

- Include more time standing, walking or cycling during your commute.

- Take the stairs rather than the lift or do a combo. Walking down stairs is just as good as walking up.

- Use a variable-height desk (with a comfort mat to reduce fatigue from standing).

- Try a wobble/balance board while working at your variable-height desk.

- Try a treadmill desk.

- Use active seating.

- Walk to your colleague's office for a face-to-face conversation rather than sending an email or text message.

- Get up at regular intervals through your day for a stretch or a walk. Set a timer on your phone if necessary.

- Hold standing or walking meetings.

Maybe you've noticed how much better you feel when you've spent more time on your feet during the day. It's disappointing to hear stories of employees being told the only way they can get a variable-height desk is if they have a note from their doctor saying they have a back problem that requires it. Isn't prevention a better, more cost-effective solution?

If your boss is yet to be convinced, they might be interested to know that having the opportunity to stand more across our working day has been associated with reports of a 71 per cent increase in focus, a 66 per cent increase in productivity, and 33 per cent less stress and fatigue. Feeling good, more alert and getting more done has to be a good outcome, right?

Being more physically active makes you more productive.

Setting your fitness goals

Start low and go slow — yes, you've heard this advice already. There are no extra brownie points for setting unrealistic targets or getting injured from overtraining. If starting from ground zero, your initial goal might be to take a 10- to 15-minute walk three times a week and to build from there. You might have set your sights on the New York Marathon, but let's get to the letterbox safely first.

Exercise building programs such as the *From Couch to 5 kms* app are a safe and fun way to start you off and keep you motivated to stretch that little bit further.

Buddying up is great for accountability. Whether it's your partner, a friend, a personal trainer or your dog, exercising in company is fun, helps to take your mind off the effort and can spark your competitive streak.

Choose your weapon

The best exercise is always the exercise you do. Remember, it's the consistency of the practice that provides the benefits, but mixing it up helps to prevent boredom and will strengthen different parts of your body. Whether you choose Tai Chi, kick boxing, water polo or kayaking, it's all about doing something you grow to enjoy and look forward to. After all, this is going to be something you will be doing for the rest of your life.

Be willing to step outside your comfort zone

Always thought you'd be terrible at tennis? Until you've given it a go, you'll never know, and even if you are, this is more about fun and participation than about qualifying for the Australian Open.

Try out different forms of exercise — there are so many options. You might like the idea of high-intensity interval training

(HIIT), with very short bursts of intense activity broken up by short intervals of rest. HIIT is ideal for time-poor executives. You may be used to concentric exercise such as biceps curls and abdominal crunches, or you might want to consider getting a little eccentric in your routine.

Eccentric exercise isn't about dressing up in fancy dress or doing weird moves. It's about movement that lengthens a muscle at the same as it is being contracted. Examples are *slooooowly* sitting down on a chair, walking down stairs, lowering an object or lying down. The benefits include increased muscle mass, balance and flexibility, improved insulin sensitivity and blood lipid profile — all without breaking a sweat.

Professor Ken Nosaka, director of exercise and sports science at Edith Cowan University, recommends eccentric exercise as the perfect resistance training for maintaining and strengthening skeletal muscles. And the cherry on the top is that it appears to have a cognitive benefit too. Why not look for ways to enjoy both?

 The best exercise routine includes eccentric and concentric exercise.

Seeking out the opportunities

What you do for exercise and when you do it will be constrained by your schedule and the types of facilities available to you.

Starting with the best intention is great, but using exercise to get into good shape mentally, physically and emotionally is going to require two things:

⚭ putting in the necessary time and effort

⚭ persevering *no matter what.*

All physical activity has value, so first look at how you get to and from work. Can you change from driving every day to cycling several times a week or doing a combination of driving and walking? If you are predominantly desk based at work, can you stand up and move around more? Try taking a minimum five-minute standing and walking break every 60 to 90 minutes.

One company I know provides its staff with walking trails of different lengths. Got 20 minutes for a meeting? Great, head for the 20-minute route trail and off you go. A variation of this is the 'walkie-talkie' meeting where you use your phone to hold the meeting, while walking around the block.

If your work naturally keeps you on your feet for much of the day, you won't need to work in as much additional exercise to meet the recommended minimum.

Your prescription for moving more

- Get off your bottom, stand up and move more at regular intervals. If you have a sedentary job or lifestyle, set an alarm on your phone to remind you to get up for a stretch or a jog around the office, or do a couple of yoga poses every 60 to 90 minutes.

- As a more upstanding citizen, look for the opportunities to stay on your feet – in meetings, at conferences, watching Netflix or on your work commute.

- When meeting a friend for coffee or lunch why not make it a 'grab and go'? Chatting while walking is fun and energising, and makes you feel good.

- Challenge your mindset. If you've always hated the idea of playing golf, surprise yourself by trying it out. You might indeed hate it, or it could turn out to be your new fun sport. Having a go is what counts.

- Flush out all those movement opportunities during your day. You may be surprised at how much you already do but didn't count, such as walking, shopping, gardening or housework. And if these activities are anathema to you, and you can afford it, pay someone else to do them to free up your time so you can go and be active in a way you do enjoy.

- Exercise for a good cause. Why not get a team together to walk, cycle or swim for charity?

- If your daily schedule makes exercising Monday to Friday an impossible challenge, try making it a normal part of your weekend.

- Take up a hobby that requires you to move; how about stand-up paddle boarding, bushwalking/rambling or Irish dancing?

- Get a grip. Grip strength reflects your cognitive capacity so get your muscles working with two sessions of resistance/weights work each week.

- Chart your progress. Build up the time you spend exercising in small increments to reach the *minimum* of 120 minutes of moderate-intensity exercise each week.

- Of all our lifestyle options exercise has the greatest capacity to keep you fit and healthy, to build greater mental wellbeing, to develop a more positive outlook and to keep you cognitively strong at every age. It's time to embrace exercise as the smartest and easiest way to stay happy and thriving.

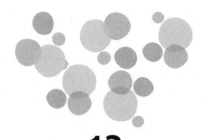

13

Music
and dance

*Getting into your groove with a jiggle and a wiggle is the
quickest, easiest and most fun way to get out of a funk
and get happy.*
J.B.

During my time at university the alternative to hanging out
in a smoky pub on a Friday night was to go to one of the local
nightclubs in the seedier end of town that held regular student
discos. The cheap entertainment was a big plus.

We girls would pile our handbags up on the floor so they
didn't get nicked, form a circle and dance around those bags
to the point of exhaustion. It was dark and the carpet horribly
sticky from goodness knows what, but it was our escape from
the drudgery of long hours of study and stress as we bopped, fist
bumped and sang along.

Dance as movement therapy

There's something quite wonderful about being able to get up and dance, confident in the knowledge that nobody's watching, like Hugh Grant dancing to the Pointer Sisters' song 'Jump (for My Love)' in the film *Love Actually*. Having a quick jiggle and wiggle around the kitchen when feeling happy is something I love to do in the sole company of our old dog, who watches disinterestedly, one eye open, from the safety of her basket.

Is dance something you incorporate into your own life, just for fun?

Watching dance can evoke powerful emotions. Sergei Polunin's interpretation of Hozier's song 'Take Me to Church', a haunting and mesmerisingly beautiful dance, quickly went viral on YouTube.

But can dance be healing? Darcey Bussell, former principal of the Royal Ballet Company in the UK, believes so. Since her retirement Dame Darcey has become an advocate for dance as a means to elevate mental wellbeing. She herself has expressed how dance helps to keep her 'on an even keel'. In a BBC documentary she shared how dance has been shown to have beneficial effects on mood and behaviour.

As one example, she followed the work of Kevin Turner, who ran a series of workshops for young people from a mental health charity in Manchester called 42nd Street, to see what impact providing a safe and creative environment would have on young people struggling with a variety of mental health issues. Encouraging these young people to express their emotions through dance produced an extraordinarily heart-warming outcome.

In her thesis 'Dancing, Mindfulness, and Our Emotions: Embracing the Mind, Body and Sole', Alisha Collins explores how dance along with mindfulness practice can be used as an intervention to better manage our emotions. Her hypothesis is that dance therapy can contribute to emotional regulation and improved mental health, building on the idea that dance, along with other creative activities including art and music, fosters resilience and wellbeing.

> **Dance can help us to express our emotions and boost our mental wellbeing.**

Dancing at any age is great

Tom, one of the participants in the Stay Sharp Community Program run in Perth, is in his early eighties and remains physically active by following a weekly schedule that includes three sessions of dancing — rock and roll, ballroom and line dancing — plus singing in a choir several times a week, and exercise that includes social tennis, a power bar gym class, Tai Chi, yoga, Pilates and an eccentric exercise class. Clearly no slouch, Tom believes being as active as possible with a variety of activities including dance is what keeps him healthy and happy, and I'm sure he's right.

If dance is something you've always fancied learning but never got around to it, now is the time — and age is never a barrier.

Designed for the over 55s, the Silver Swans ballet classes are now a global phenomenon introducing older learners to ballet dancing, with all ages and abilities catered for. A 55-minute session to enhance flexibility, posture and coordination while feeling as graceful as a swan sounds highly appealing, non-threatening and, importantly, fun!

A study published in the journal *Frontiers of Human Neuroscience* showed how of all the physical activities we take part in to retain our cognition as we age, dance has the most profound effect on the hippocampus, assisting in maintaining our memory, learning and balance. The lead researcher Kathrin Rehfeld observed how 'exercise has the beneficial effect of slowing down or counteracting age-related decline in mental and physical capacity'.

Good news for all of us, especially if you're anticipating staying longer in the workforce because you want to keep contributing usefully.

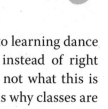

Dance is a fantastic way to cross-train the brain because it requires all our skills – mental, physical, emotional and social.

If like me you have two left feet when it comes to learning dance moves (I was always the one who went left instead of right when following my aerobics instructor), that's not what this is about. Your current ability is irrelevant, which is why classes are good for helping us improve! Practice and repetition allow your natural neuroplasticity to embed new neural pathways. Feeling good with dance is possible for all of us.

It can feel hard to find (or make) the time to add something like dance lessons to our schedule. We get too caught up with other activities like taking the kids to all their out-of-school activities. But when it comes to signing up for a weekly dance class of some sort, there's no reason why we shouldn't (other than the excuses of being time poor and talentless) and every reason why we should. Learning to express yourself through dance improves coordination, general fitness and confidence, which is why it is sometimes incorporated into psychological counselling.

Taking up some form of dance adds to our bucket of positive emotion, and when done in a group the delight is contagious. So, as Justin Timberlake reminds us in his song 'Can't Stop the Feeling', let's just dance. It's hard *not* to move when grooving to a song that makes us feel happy.

Getting into dance groove at work

If the thought of dancing at work sounds too ridiculous, bear in mind that it's been shown to assist in team building, communication, problem solving, and building confidence, energy and creativity. And it makes us smarter by enhancing neuroplasticity. According to Stanford University's Richard Powers, in his article 'Use It or Lose It: Dancing Makes You Smarter, Longer', 'Dancing integrates several brain functions at once — kinesthetic, rational, musical, and emotional — further increasing your neural connectivity.'

Companies such as John Lewis and Utilita in the UK have promoted flash mob performances that boost everyone's mood. Running an in-house competition for best dance can be fun too. No matter what our job description, dancing unites us all.

Move It Monday is an international campaign encouraging people of all fitness levels to get moving each week, starting on Monday (when else?), because it's such a great stress buster, and doing dancerise is easy. Just put on your headphones and dance your way to happiness. Improv, rap, tap or swing, it's your choice. Time to put on your dancing shoes.

Let the music play

What role does music play in your life? Are you a not-so-secret singer in the shower, an air guitar player extraordinaire or someone who likes to sing along to all your favourite songs safe in the soundproof vault of your car? Which feel-good tracks do you choose to sand blast your ear-drums at full volume?

Whether we're being 'Happy' with Pharrell Williams, humming along to the *Game of Thrones* soundtrack or entranced by Samuel Barber's deeply moving *Adagio for Strings*, our familiarity with the music instantly transports us into a certain mental state. It changes how we see the world.

Music can transport us to a joyful and happy space.

The brainy benefits of music

Music has always been with us in one form or another across the millennia. It's believed to have contributed to the development of human speech and it activates almost every region of the brain. It's capable of triggering long-forgotten memories, bringing us to tears and inspiring great joy.

In her TEDx talk music educator Anita Collins makes the point that music is a complete workout for the brain, engaging multiple areas including the motor, sensory visual, prefrontal and auditory cortices, and the cerebellum.

Scientific studies have shown that music plays an important role in influencing our emotional state as well as our ability to learn, to stay on task, to use our higher thinking skills and to be more creative.

A small study in Germany showed that listening to classical music by composers such as Wagner and Strauss decreases blood pressure and lowers cortisol levels while boosting the release of dopamine, which also has a modulating effect on stress, so we feel more relaxed.

Listening to music we enjoy triggers our brain's reward circuitry, leading to an increase in the amount of dopamine released. Neuroscientist Daniel Levitin, author of *This Is Your Brain on Music*, talks about how music triggers our anticipation of what comes next, boosting our level of dopamine, which is why we enjoy singing along to our favourite songs so much.

Music triggers powerful memories

Music plays an enormously important role in our lives, irrespective of our own musical abilities, connecting us at a deeper level to past events or memories, which is why we get teary or happy when we hear a certain song or choose to belt out the chorus of our favourite tune when driving to work. That introductory riff that is so familiar immediately takes us back to the rock concert, holiday or people we were with when we last, or first, heard it.

 Music helps us tap into those emotions we often are very good at burying deep.

Music is a very powerful memory trigger, because memory and music perception use the same neural circuitry, which is why 'Singing for the Brain' groups work so well in providing emotional support for those living with dementia. A person may have lost the ability to communicate coherently, but hearing a familiar song triggers the memory, which allows them to sing along word perfect.

Music for mental wellbeing

Do you ever use music to give you a boost? Meta reviews of the scientific literature have revealed the positive impact of music on depression, anxiety and pain. The British Academy for Sound Therapy recommends 78 minutes (very precise!) as a daily minimum for mental wellbeing, while the US National Institutes of Health has funded US$20 million for a sound health initiative to investigate where music can be a useful intervention to promote wellbeing across a range of medical conditions.

Music has also been shown to be effective in modulating chronic pain. Jymmin is a training concept that combines a workout using a fitness machine with free musical improvisation. It's been shown to help those exercising to reach their physical activity goals with less effort and also improves motivation and mood. Even without pain, exercising to music helps us to maintain a faster tempo and keeps us going for longer.

Being continually exposed to ambient noise in cities — traffic, air-conditioners, aeroplanes, jackhammers, sirens and so on — has been shown to adversely affect our heath, elevating rates of heart disease, high blood pressure, obesity, poor sleep and lower mood. It sounds like a good time to consider using music as a way of diminishing the impact of noise pollution on our health.

If you listened to more music in the past than you do now, what would rekindle that pleasure and interest?

Music is a connector

Neuroscientist and musician Alan Harvey describes music as 'a social glue that enhances our sense of mental wellbeing'. Oliver Sacks calls our love of producing and listening to music 'musicophilia'. Of course we are not all gifted musicians, and fortunately most of us recognise our own shortcomings before choosing to audition for *The Voice*. I'd always fancied learning how to sing better and join a choir, so I enrolled in a course aptly called 'Singing for non-Singers'. It was hilarious (we were quite bad!), but it also taught us a very important thing: our self-limiting beliefs around our abilities too often hold us back and close us off from activities that could bring us great joy. There's something magical that happens when you sing in a group. Your heart rates synchronise and you become as one, regardless of capability.

Tania de Jong AM has been running the choirs 'With One Voice' since 2008, bringing together people from diverse backgrounds and cultures to promote social inclusion and creativity. For her the biggest bonus is in witnessing the increases in self-belief, confidence, joy and ability to cope with life's challenges. She sees it as a way of dealing more effectively with our distracted and frenetic lives, boosting endorphins, dopamine and oxytocin, which make us feel happy, healthy and rewarded.

Recent research has shown how singing for one hour can boost levels of immune proteins in people diagnosed with cancer, lowering stress, improving mood and supporting greater mental wellbeing.

Singing makes us happy, *especially* when we're in a group. Which is why one group of researchers are looking at the use of group singing as an adjunct treatment for those suffering anxiety and depression.

Music at work

Do you listen to music while you work?

When our children were teenagers a common evening difference of opinion (read argument) in our household was over the perennial issue of listening to music while doing homework. My view, no doubt influenced by my personality and past experience of being lectured on the importance of a quiet environment when studying, was against it, while our children railed against the parental diktat, insisting they studied better when listening to their favourite songs.

As a junior doctor working as a surgical intern, I noted how some surgeons preferred to operate listening to music (or in some instances the cricket) while deeply absorbed in their painstaking work, though this certainly didn't indicate they weren't paying attention to what else was going on. 'Pull back harder on that retractor, Brockis. And stop shuffling your feet!'

In workshops I often like to play a little background music while participants are busy working on a group activity.

So who is on the right side of this argument? It depends on the individual, their emotional state and the environment. If you're feeling stressed or anxious, listening to something you find calming can be beneficial. For high-performing individuals such as surgeons, reducing stress and the associated emotions can serve to improve concentration and focus.

It's also good for the patient! Listening to relaxing music before undergoing a procedure has been shown to be effective in reducing anxiety and may even be used as an alternative to sedation.

People working in highly creative environments, such as software developers, have been shown to work faster and more effectively when listening to music, remaining more aware of what is going on around them, more highly engaged and curious. The performance of these individuals actually drops when the music is turned off.

In one office-based experiment, neuropsychologist David Lewis reported that 88 per cent of participants were found to produce their most accurate test results when listening to music. The speed of work appears to depend on the genre of music played and the type of work being undertaken.

It was found that:

- pop music is best when the need is to work quickly and accurately
- classical music is most effective when grappling with mathematical problems
- ambient music improves data entry accuracy (perhaps by mitigating the boredom effect)
- dance music was great for improving proofreading.

The experiment's overall results showed that nine out of ten people performed better when listening to music, reporting a positive influence on morale, motivation and output. Given the choice of four different genres to listen to, 81 per cent of participants worked faster when listening to music.

We are all different, of course, and while the evidence suggests music can have a useful place in the workplace, it's important to take into account individual differences in personality and personal choice, and the complexity of the tasks being undertaken.

Music can boost productivity at work.

Have you got your own personal playlist for work?

In their book *Your Playlist Can Change Your Life: 10 Proven Ways Your Favorite Music Can Revolutionize Your Health, Memory, Organization, Alertness and More*, Mindlin, DuRousseau and Cardillo explain how 'next to the sense of smell, your musical choice produces an immediate impact to influence and reset your brain networks without the need for any external substance or drug'. Coffee or music or both? What works for you?

Choosing your playlist is about seeking out those songs that you find uplifting and inspirational and that promote a state of flow. Try playing your list on the way to work, before settling in for your working day, and work towards creating a set of different lists to suit your mood and the work you'll be engaged in.

It's clear that music can change our brains and us for the better. Not only that, it's inspiring and fun.

Your prescription for adding more dance and music to your life

- If music has always been an important part of your life, how can you use it now to consciously lift your mood, boost your productivity *and* extend your musical repertoire?

- Set yourself up for a great day by playing some music you like with a little jiggle and wiggle as you get up in the morning. Classical can be calming, pop music more upbeat.

(continued)

- Turn on the radio or the app on your phone while on your commute to work. Choose music you find energising (or calming, especially if driving in peak-hour traffic drives you nuts). Using music to reduce the risk of road rage can make the school drop-off and the search for that elusive parking spot at work so much less stressful.

- If it's been a while since you put on your dancing shoes, make the decision to reintroduce dance and music into your life. Sign up for a dance class, join a choir or book tickets for a concert.

- If there's a clarinet, guitar or saxophone that's been quietly gathering dust in the back of the cupboard, why not get it out and surprise yourself at how your fingers (kind of) remember what to do. It's a great way to stimulate your happiness and wellbeing – okay, and maybe a little frustrating initially when you realise just how rusty you've become. But that neural memory will still be there and, just like riding a bike, will come back quickly given the opportunity and practice.

- Explore using music at work to boost your performance and productivity. Using headphones (when appropriate) means you won't be imposing your musical preferences on others.

- Give yourself permission to hang loose. Whether or not you did ballet as a child or loved gyrating to pop songs as a teenager, giving yourself permission to get a little more flexible and shake out all that muscle tension is a great way to limber up. Worried about looking silly? We can all look a little ridiculous when dancing. Have you ever watched people dance at a silent disco? Ridiculousness is super cool because it allows you to express who you are.

- Join the vinyl revival. Whether you're old enough to have your own vintage collection from the last century or just starting out, spending time listening to music from different eras or genres will stretch your mental muscles and provide you with a new appreciation of how music has played such an important role in our social and emotional evolution. Which reminds me, it's time I reclaimed my Bob Dylan album from my brother.

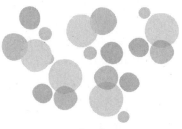

14

Blue and green – complete the scene

I go to nature to be soothed, healed and have my senses put in order.
John Burroughs

Our wellbeing is intrinsically bound up with the world around us. It's time to remember our place in the world's ecosystem and how our environment has shaped our evolutionary path. Which is why we often feel so much better when we've spent time in nature. It's good for our body, mind and soul, and now we have the science to back this up.

Moving to Australia from the UK, where the norm was low grey cloud accompanied by mizzle, drizzle or incessant rain, I couldn't get enough of waking up to yet another day of clear blue skies, sunshine and warmth.

Have you noticed how obsessed we are with the weather? We all talk about it. Constantly. Maybe we're finding it too hot, or too cold, too dry or too wet — or just perfect. Everyone has an opinion on this subject they want to share. Will the weather be good for the upcoming cricket match, the barbie you're hosting on the weekend or your wedding next week?

Whether it's that favourite park bench where you like to eat your lunch, or picking a desk close to a window with an outlook, or one with high ceilings, loads of natural light and indoor plants, nature impacts your work life in any number of ways each day, influencing your mood, attention and general wellbeing.

If you're fed up sitting in an airless, gloomy box that's either an oven or a deep freeze because the central system controls the whole building and doesn't allow for individual variability, it's time to go green.

One of the most challenging workplaces I've ever had to work in as a GP was a small windowless office in a suburban practice that had just enough room for the examination couch, a table and two chairs. The flickering fluorescent tube cast a sterile and unwelcoming light. I understood how Harry must have felt living in his cupboard under the stairs, though I bet he never had the challenge of what to do when the power went off while in the middle of undertaking a well-woman check. Y*es, that well-woman check!*

With no outlook and not a skerrick of green to relieve the sterile setting, I never knew if it was sunny or snowing outside (though the latter would have been somewhat unlikely in Perth). A pot plant, though it would have had to be a small one to fit into that ridiculously small space, could have made a difference for both the doctor and her patients. As it was, it was deeply depressing.

We need to get out more

Estimates put the average amount of time we now spend indoors at 80 to 95 per cent. If you find that hard to credit, take a moment to estimate how much time you spend indoors on an average day. The result may surprise you.

What has been called our 'nature deficit' recognises the amount of time we're spending indoors, online and disconnected from the healing power of nature to buffer us against the stresses of modern life.

In *Your Brain on Nature*, co-author Alan Logan argues that being in nature is about more than just helping to reduce our stress; it enhances our vitality. He sees one of the principal reasons we don't spend more time in nature as being because we are 'time crunched'. Our sense of time poverty is one of a number of lifestyle choices, including our dependence on technology, that are among the chief causes of our alienation from nature. The paradox is that the research shows how staying in nature helps us to reclaim the sense of having enough time.

Little wonder one of the emerging trends shaping the US$4.2 trillion wellness industry outlined in the annual Global Wellness Summit is the prescription of nature as a medicine.

Prescribing nature is a new wellness trend.

The brainy benefits of spending time in nature

Have you heard? Experiencing nature protects our mental and physical wellbeing. It's recommended that we spend a minimum of 120 minutes outdoors each week. This was one of the findings of a research study undertaken at the University of Exeter where survey data from 20 000 people showed this to be the threshold above which people were more likely to report good health and better mental wellbeing. This holds true for men and women of different ages and different socioeconomic and ethnic backgrounds, and even those living with illness or disability.

Living in or close to a green urban space is known to be linked to lower rates of heart disease, obesity, diabetes, mental distress and mortality, better self-reported health, subjective wellbeing, birth outcomes and cognitive development, and lower rates of myopia (short-sightedness) in children. Living in a green urban space or taking time out to visit local parks contributes significantly to helping you keep things in perspective.

 Twenty minutes outside in a green space is enough to lower the amount of the stress hormone cortisol in your system.

The idea of turning to nature to lower stress is not new. The Japanese have engaged with forest bathing or Shinrin–Yoku since 1982. This has nothing to do with bathing or water; rather, it's about slowing down to take a gentle stroll in a forest setting. Consciously taking in your surroundings engages all your senses. It becomes a form of meditative practice.

Think of times you have stood on top of a hill to take in a country view, paused to listen to the sound of birdsong or the wind in the trees, or blessed silence, or marvelled at the power of the elements while watching the waves crash on the shore, and you have felt a deeper sense of connection, of wonder and awe. Psychologist Professor Dacher Keltner at UCLA Berkeley describes the feeling of being present in something vast that transcends our understanding of the world, stimulating a sense of wonder and curiosity. And this sense of awe in nature can be transformative.

Taking time out for such activities promotes reflection and introspection, leading to more divergent thought, which is why a long weekend in the country or attending a retreat or simply going for a long beach or bush walk can be so beneficial. Simply being more physically active brings the extra benefit of raising dopamine and serotonin levels, elevating mood and boosting the immune system.

This is not the time for selfies or Instagram pics. Switch off your phone and choose to enjoy feeling good while benefiting from lower stress, lower blood pressure and improved cardiac and lung function.

Ecotherapy, as it's called, is increasingly practised in Japan, Australia and the UK to treat anxiety and depression.

 Forest bathing is a great way to reduce stress.

Go Dutch to clear your head

Remember that bracing walk along the coastal path or mountain trail and how energised as well as windswept you felt. Blowing out those cobwebs is something the Dutch love to do. They use such windy exercise, which they call *uitwaaien*, to clear the mind and elevate their sense of wellbeing.

There's something else blowing in the wind too. It's the smell: pine trees or eucalypts, or the dank decomposition of the rainforest floor all contribute to our sensory experience of being in nature. What's more, trees and plants release what are called phytoncides, which protect them from insects and germs but have also been shown to boost the human immune system, increase anticancer protein production, reduce stress, improve mood and basically make us feel good. Cedar and cypress phytoncide has been shown to be calming and a great immune system booster.

So let's breathe in a few more phytoncides now.

It's calming

Have you ever wondered why your dentist gets you to watch those endless replays of *The Blue Planet* on the TV monitor hovering over your head? They know that distracting you this way takes your mind off a potentially unpleasant procedure, especially when you're going to be in that chair for a bit while you have a crown fixed or that filling done. (Thankfully we have moved on from the days when the fish tank in the waiting room and a stack of ancient, over-thumbed copies of *National Geographic* offered the only diversion.)

Which begs the question, is it better to spend time in a green or a blue space? They are probably of equal value, and which you favour may depend on where you live. Blue is our most popular colour, and water has long been associated with healing and relaxing qualities.

According to marine biologist Wallace J. Nichols, author of *Blue Mind*, spending any amount of time 'near, in, on or under water' increases our wellbeing and happiness.

Living close to water, whether the sea, a river or lake, or a village pond, is associated with higher levels of physical activity (around 30 minutes more exercise per week), lower stress and a reduced risk of psychological distress. If you have a green or blue space nearby it's easier to find the time for that extra outdoor exercise, which is also more appealing. You'll have more opportunities to enjoy picnics with your partner, family or friends, or to stretch your legs with a walk, hike or cycle ride, with the bonus of better air quality.

The outcome? A greater ability to cope with life's challenges and a lower mortality rate. No wonder real estate with blue or green views commands premium prices.

Initiatives such as the UK's Blue Health 2020 Project, which explores the best ways city dwellers can take advantage of blue space to improve wellbeing, can help us all counteract the high levels of stress and overwhelm of modern life.

Whether you love watching the waves crashing on the beach in a storm, or swimming in or walking along the river, a watery environment engages all your senses. The feel of the sand between your toes, the smell of salt and seaweed, the sound of water over rocks, a blue vista or a gentle river current triggers a positive cascade of biochemical responses.

Nichols suggests even taking a shower can have a calming effect on our mind, washing away stress and anxieties. Perhaps that's why we come up with some of our best insights in the shower and find soaking in a hot tub so relaxing. It allows us to disconnect from our worries and reconnect with what's important. Anyone for an *onsen*?

Over recent years float tanks have become increasingly popular, promoted as a way to detoxify from the stresses of life, creating deep relaxation by inducing a daydreamy state of more theta brain waves. While I've yet to sample the delight of lying naked in a dark tank, people I know who've tried it say it made them feel great.

Swimming can also feel meditative, whether you're following that black line in the pool or stroking your way between two groynes off the beach. One colleague shared how whenever she's faced with a particularly challenging problem, she goes for a swim to clear her mind and find the solution she seeks more easily. This works by taking our focus away from our dominant left hemisphere, which is trying to nail down a logical, analytical solution, and activating the brain's default-mode network to gain access to more insightful and creative ideas. Why not try it and see if it works for you?

 Spending time in a blue or green space is good for our physical and mental wellbeing.

It makes you happier, boosts cognition and increases longevity

Stanford researcher Gregory Bratman has shown how taking a 90-minute walk in nature rather than an urban environment helps to reduce rumination — the mental activity where you get caught up in endless worrying — by decreasing activity in the part of the brain associated with this type of thinking, the subgenual prefrontal cortex, which can lead to an increased risk of depression.

He also showed that strolling through a green environment has a more positive effect in boosting attention and happiness than walking for the same length of time in an area of heavy traffic.

Data from the Nurses' Health Study, a series of prospective studies examining the epidemiology and long-term effects of nutrition, hormones, environment and work–life balance, showed how women living in greener areas had a 12 per cent lower mortality rate compared with those with less exposure to green space. Another, small study of 20 people with diagnosed clinical depression, showed how getting out for a walk in the park also provided cognitive benefits, boosting working memory and attention.

Growing up in a green area has been shown to boost curiosity and engagement in children, skills that will surely benefit them as they grow up.

It restores attention

If you've ever found yourself desperate for inspiration or struggling to stay on task, nature can help. Working in front of a computer screen for any length of time quickly exhausts the brain, increasing stress and contributing to a sense of time passing too quickly.

This is where taking a 40-second break to look out of the office window onto a green space — whether a tree-lined street or green city roof — will help to restore your focus. Having a pot plant either on your desk or at least in your field of vision helps to achieve the same thing.

Exposure to greenery helps reduce our attention deficit and overcome attention fatigue, while increasing our creativity and problem-solving ability.

If your much-maligned office pot plant is looking a tad dusty and neglected, it's probably time to seek out new green ways to boost your productivity and wellbeing. Studies have shown that enriching the workplace environment with growing plants increases workplace satisfaction, self-reported levels of concentration and perceived air quality over the short and longer term.

The COGfx studies from Harvard and Syracuse Universities and UTC found that US 'green certified' offices reported a 25 per cent increase in cognition, a 33 per cent lower absenteeism rate and a 6 per cent increase in reported sleep quality. Does your workplace need to get certified? But 'green office design', which is about designing environmentally to humanise the workplace, can go one step further by adding greenery to boost productivity by a further 15 per cent. The University of Exeter showed how adding plants to the office space raises engagement, concentration and perceived air quality.

What all this is telling us is that connecting with nature can really benefit our health. Green or blue, it's up to you.

Greening up your day, week, month, year

While moving house or office might not be an option, there are a number of other ways you can work towards reducing your nature deficit.

Check out where the green spaces are in your locality

It's not uncommon to discover that because you take the same route to work every day and go to the same places over the weekend, you've been missing out on an amazing park, wetland or inner-city green space around the corner you didn't know existed.

Look for ways to increase the time you spend outside each day

Is it practical to get outside for lunch or to add in a 20- or 30-minute walk or jog during your lunchbreak? Can you shake up your commute? Are there any other greener alternatives you could add to your 120 minutes of outside time?

Sign up for an eduventure

A number of companies now offer eduventures and walks to boost creativity, reduce stress and enhance wellbeing. In Australia, Wild Women on Top is an organisation that focuses on women's health and wellbeing through shared hiking adventures and walks. Their charity arm, Coastrek, raises money for mental health. Edgewalkers in West Australia take small groups on walking tours using nature to stimulate participants' creative potential. Great if you're planning on writing a book!

Make the time

If time is the issue, start with five minutes.

Jules Pretty, Professor of Environment and Society at the University of Exeter, believes as little as five minutes outdoors can have a positive impact on our mood, sense of self-worth and identity. It's powerful stuff and is always on tap. And it costs nothing except your time and willingness to participate.

Making the time is one of our biggest hurdles. You may have a state forest on your doorstep or live close to the beach, but how often do you take advantage of it?

Add in more greenery at home and work

You may not have a green thumb (I can relate to this, having once managed to kill the almost indestructible cheese plant), but there are loads of water-wise, low-maintenance plants that you can set and forget. Speak to your local nursery experts, who can give you plenty of advice.

If your workplace has an anti-green policy, even an image will help. A good photo or print of a beautiful green space is a good start. Remember this is about your health and wellbeing, not just a means to hide that ugly piece of office furniture.

Your prescription to reduce your nature deficit

- Aim to get outside every day for at least 20 to 30 minutes or a minimum of two hours a week.

- Choose activity over passivity – get up and get out.

- Take back control of your time and choose to do something that makes you feel good in the great outdoors. Start gardening or mountain biking or join a walking group. Maybe bird watching or ocean swimming is more your style.

- Use walking as a means to avoid waiting! If hanging around is driving you nuts or worry is getting you down, getting outside for a short walk can help restore calm and peace of mind.

- Buy some pot plants for the patio, balcony or office, or create a living wall or a roof garden.

- Go for a swim in the ocean (if nearby) or an outside pool. Seek out green and blue destinations and start visiting them regularly.

- Establish a new routine such as going for a walk after work or after dinner.

Part IV

Human

Hard-wired to connect

We are like islands in the sea, separate on the surface but connected in the deep.
William James

Elinor and I have been best friends for the best part of forty years. We met at medical school and just 'clicked'. We've been housemates together, have always celebrated and commiserated our various triumphs and failures together and supported each other during challenging times. She was bridesmaid at our wedding and is godmother to our daughter. Others have sometimes mistaken us for sisters because we're alike in so many ways. Once left alone in a room we can talk and laugh together for hours, picking up from our last conversation as if it was five minutes ago. Our bond is as strong today as it's ever been, despite the fact we live on opposite sides of the world.

Relationships matter, and in a world that can sometimes be cruel, violent and judgemental there's never been a greater need for more human connection.

 It's the strength of our interpersonal relationships that keeps us safe, healthy and happy.

Wired to connect

Being a member of the *Homo sapiens* species puts you in a pretty special group. You're capable not just of thinking but of knowing how to regulate your emotions and build a network of relationships.

From an evolutionary perspective, belonging to a group meant being able to:

- learn new skills more quickly through the sharing of information and ideas

- ⚡ stay safe from predators, so long as you abide by the tribal rules, don't get too big for your boots or try to take over the leadership

- ⚡ contribute to the continuing success of the species by finding a mate and undertaking a spot of procreation.

We operate within a number of different group or tribal contexts, including family, friends and work colleagues, each with its own set of conventions and rules. While building your emotional intelligence is great, understanding more about your social brain and how it works to sustain stronger positive relationships is vital to your physical and mental wellbeing and overall happiness.

Connection allows us to survive and thrive

Social cognitive behavioural neuroscientist Professor Matt Lieberman believes our ability to form relationships is as important to our survival as the food, air and water we need. If you think about it, this makes perfect sense. Human babies are born functionally immature, unable to care for themselves, totally dependent on a caregiver for safety and sustenance. Which is why a new mother's brain pumps out massive amounts of the bonding chemical oxytocin to help her connect with this pink squirming bundle of joy she has just brought into the world.

Being social is an obsession

We crave social approval and because we care so much about what other people think (what, you mean that's not true for you?), our actions and behaviour are heavily influenced by how we think others may see us. Meaning that in *any* social situation our brain is asking questions like, 'Am I accepted? Is it safe to be here, and if so where's my reward?'

The payoff is that a sense of belonging makes us happy.

How this works is that at any given moment when your brain isn't actively focused, it switches to what is called your default mode network (DMN), which evolved to help us learn about our social environment. Why? Matt Lieberman proposes that 'evolution made a bet that the best thing for a brain to do in any spare moment is to get ready for what comes next in social terms'.

Our need to belong

Whether at work or in our friendships and close relationships, a sense of belonging makes us feel safe, which is great. The flipside, though, is that if you feel that no matter how hard you try you're just not fitting in, that you're on the outer and not part of the group, it can lead to a sense of disconnect and social pain. Rejection hurts.

Social pain is real

Denied the pleasure of feeling included and cared about, the social pain of exclusion wounds. If you've experienced a relationship break-up, or faced disapproval from a family member, or been criticised at work, you may have used words such as, 'It broke my heart', 'I feel gutted' or 'It was a real kick in the guts'. We use the language of physical pain, which should come as no surprise as experiencing social pain activates similar areas in the brain as physical pain.

Understanding just how painful, deep and long-lasting social pain can be matters because it's typically invisible, hidden from view. In this sense, social pain is more like a soft tissue injury than breaking a bone. A hamstring injury can take longer to recover from than a fractured femur. Telling someone to 'suck it up' after being berated for some wrongdoing or 'You'll get over it — there are plenty more fish in the sea!' when experiencing heartbreak at best is unhelpful and at worst adds to the pain already felt.

You could try taking a couple of Tylenol, but despite studies suggesting it can help reduce the intensity of social pain, I don't recommend you propose it when offering consolation to others; they might not take it in the way you intended.

 Social pain hurts as much as physical pain because they share common neural pathways.

You can experience social pain when:

- your name has been missed off an email invitation to an important meeting about a project you've been working on for the past six months

- you notice your colleagues' rolled eyes or raised eyebrows as you stand to present your thoughts when answering a question in a meeting

- you feel excluded from the group conversation taking place in the lunch queue — you are being quietly outed

- you overhear your name being mentioned in the context of a project you've been involved with, and the comments aren't flattering

- an anonymous troll posts an unkind comment or snide remark on your social media.

Social pain is a threat to our health and wellbeing. You may know someone who never fully recovered from a relationship breakdown, or from being ousted from their job for being a whistle-blower. Perhaps you've been that person.

Getting the measure of social pain

How does rejection make you feel? Whether experienced directly in person or online, social rejection triggers a massive threat response in the brain, as demonstrated by neuroscientists Eisenberger and Lieberman in their classic Cyberball experiment using fMRI to examine the impact of social exclusion.

If you're not familiar with Cyberball, here's how it works. Take one hapless human and tell them they will be playing a game of Cyberball with two other players while having their brain activity monitored as a virtual ball is tossed between the three players. It's rigged, of course. The other players are not human but part of a computer program. All goes well until the computer figures stop throwing the ball to the human.

In the debrief afterwards, the researchers were surprised by the depth of the feeling of rejection expressed by the participants, even when they had been told it was a computer they had been playing against.

A strong social network acts as a buffer that helps keep you safe from social pain. If you've made a bad mistake and your manager isn't happy with you, and has told everyone in the office of the error of your ways, knowing you still have the support of your colleagues can reduce your sense of humiliation.

The paradox of technology and connection

Oh boy, do we love to connect on our social media channels. Whether you're on Facebook, Instagram or WhatsApp, you're only a click away from making a new connection or strengthening an existing network. How brilliant to be able to hook up using Facetime, Zoom or Skype to chat with friends and colleagues anytime, anywhere.

Beyond work, our new technologies have forever changed how we look for love or make new friends. The question of the moment now is should you swipe to the left or to the right, but naturally your friends are eager to help you with the process.

The double-edged sword is that while technology is brilliant for helping you connect, the inevitable subsequent social comparisons that lead you to feel you aren't as happy, perfect or successful as your online 'friends' can produce a sense of disconnect, lower self-esteem and raise anxiety.

And then there's loneliness

The pain of loneliness or friendlessness makes us sad, and sadness is the longest lasting of all our emotions. It drives a deep longing to overcome our distress, but it can be challenging to know how to make the nights pass more quickly and those days devoid of meaningful human contact more bearable. Failing to notice the pain or hurt experienced by a friend or colleague means missing the essential cues that this is the time to show empathy and compassion and give them a big hug.

 The greatest risk of feeling disconnected is increased social isolation and loneliness.

When dealing with your own social pain, you might, depending on your personality, decide to:

- tell them how it is — how dare they treat you this way!
- simmer on a low heat, brooding on your pain, until one day you boil over
- plan your revenge for a later date by ghosting or using other well-honed passive-aggressive techniques
- withdraw silently to your cave to lick your wounds.

Beware the passive aggressor, who may torment you for years over the pain you caused them. Because they never speak openly about it, you're unaware of their hurt and left wondering why your former friend started behaving unkindly or cut you out of their social network.

Fixing social pain requires acceptance and forgiveness. Much will depend on the severity of the social breach and the strength of your previous relationship.

With connection comes trust, compassion and empathy, those unique traits that bind us as humans so we feel cared for and care about each other. It keeps us feeling safe and rewarded.

 Connection allows us to care for ourselves as well as each other.

It's time to connect and show you care

This is about:

- caring about those we love, and who we know love us

- caring about our friends, supporting them through the good times and the bad

- caring about and looking out for our colleagues, contributing to the creation of more positive and thriving workplaces.

Care isn't hard, but sometimes we need a gentle reminder. It's often the smallest of gestures that can have the biggest impact on your life, sense of connection and happiness.

Caring at the human level requires an understanding of the individual, a determination to support them in a difficult situation and a willingness to get others involved to help solve a problem.

Case Study

My friend Clare had been going through a rough patch. Her marriage had broken down and she was now a single mum with two small boys, trying to hold down a full-time job with little immediate social support as her parents and siblings lived interstate.

Not wishing to be a burden on her colleagues, and terrified of losing her job, she hadn't told her boss of the change in her circumstances and had only confided in one friend at work. Seeing how fragile Clare was, her friend urged her to speak out, but she chose to stay silent. After several weeks of watching her friend struggle, seeing the dark rings around her eyes from lack of sleep and the clear evidence that she wasn't coping, she told Clare she couldn't stand by any longer and was going to speak to their boss.

Later that afternoon Clare's boss called her into his office to discuss new arrangements that would provide her with greater flexibility in managing the school drop-offs and pick-ups, and the option of working from home one or two days a week. Knowing she was cared for and supported in this way gave Clare the confidence boost she needed to get back on track emotionally and mentally and move forward.

 The greatest gift we can ever give another human being is the gift of caring.

In these last three chapters we'll examine what helps us to connect and care for each other, because everything gets so much better when we do.

The Train of Human Connection

Buy your tickets now to jump on the train for greater connection.

- Carriage 1: There's plenty of space here for nurturing greater trust and respect.

- Carriage 2: Roll up, roll up to expand your conscious contribution to greater kindness and compassion.

- Carriage 3: With empathy in tow, oh the places you can go.

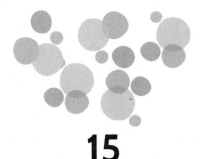

15

Trust
and respect

I am in a very unsettled condition, as the oyster said when they
poured melted butter all over his back.
Edward Lear

'You can choose to do nothing but you'll end up in a wheelchair, or you can have surgery. That carries its own risks, but there's a good chance it will alleviate your pain, prevent further nerve damage and allow you to get on with your life.'

The thought of ending up in a wheelchair was enough for my husband to agree to undergo neurosurgery on his neck. The big decision was who should do the operation? After seeking the opinion of a respected neurosurgeon and talking with him at length about the pros and cons of what would undoubtedly be a high-risk procedure, he made his decision. He left the consultation confident he could trust the surgeon he had chosen to do the best job.

Intuitively we know just how much trust matters. It determines who we will consent to remove our child's tonsils or to service our car, or which employer we will stick with. As the foundation of all relationships, trust is the social glue that binds us to partners, friends and colleagues. We value it and mourn its loss.

Trust gives you confidence and faith in the reliability, integrity and honesty of another person or entity. When someone you trust tells you they'll show up at 11 am you are confident they will. When a trusted colleague tells you they can handle their side of the project and deliver on time, you know you can relax because you take them at their word.

One of your brain's primary organising principles is *safety first, then find the reward*. As a social being, your trusted relationships enable you to prosper and grow. Feeling trusted and trusting your colleagues makes it so much easier for you to work well together. When the culture is one based on trust, you want to collaborate, contribute and be an effective team member. Trust builds loyalty and respect, reduces stress, breaks down silos and has been shown to be important to ethical decision making.

How we measure trust

At the individual level we rely on observable behaviours. At the institutional level we draw confidence from other sources. Over the past 20 years the Edelman Trust Barometer has provided an index of trust (or the lack of it) in business, government, NGOs and the media. It has shown that distrust of institutions is being driven by a growing sense of inequity and the perception that institutions are increasingly serving the interests of the powerful few over everyone else.

Add to that the concern held by 83 per cent of those surveyed that their job security is at risk, the high level of uncertainty is further threatening trust 'in the system'.

Following a depressing trend of diminishing trust, in 2019 the barometer detected one positive shift—a rise in trust between employees and employer. Why? Because it's the closest relationship that can forge change. If as an individual you feel unable to bring about positive change, you'll typically turn to the closest person in authority you believe can.

This is reflected in the statistics indicating that '58% of general population employees look to their employer to be a trustworthy source of information about contentious issues, with 71% indicating they want their CEO to respond to challenging times'. This is an invitation for strong leadership to provide greater certainty in an uncertain world and bring about the change we want to see.

The brainy benefits of trust

Trust is the foundation of all our relationships and vital to our physical health, mental wellbeing and happiness.

Trust brings happiness

Trust is a two-way street. You are more likely to trust someone when you yourself feel trusted. Then you both feel good and the relationship is strengthened. Trust allows happiness to bloom.

Chemically, this works through the neuropeptide oxytocin, which is believed to be important in establishing trust and boosting our sense of wellbeing. The release of oxytocin acts as a signal indicating 'It's safe to approach'.

Trust elevates wellbeing and longevity

Research by Duke University found people aged 55 to 80 who enjoy higher levels of interpersonal trust on average live 14 years longer. Why? If you're in a trusting relationship you're more likely to engage in social interaction, which boosts mood, lowers stress and provides greater social and emotional support.

A meta-analytical review across 148 studies found that the influence of our social relationships on our mortality is of comparable strength to that of risk factors such as smoking and alcohol consumption, and is greater than the risk of physical inactivity or obesity. This supports a research finding reported in the scientific journal *Science* back in the late eighties that, 'Social relationships, or the relative lack thereof, constitute a major risk factor for health — rivalling the effect of well-established health risk factors such as cigarette smoking, blood pressure, blood lipids, obesity and physical activity'.

These conclusions provide a strong indicator of the need to take our social relationships seriously to combat the growing tide of loneliness.

Now you know that getting to know your neighbours and maintaining good relationships with them is good for your health, perhaps it's time to get over that long-standing dispute about the fence. For the same reason it will pay to get to know your work colleagues better, especially the ones you feel less aligned to. Increasing your connection could begin by striking up a conversation in the coffee queue, starting a meeting with a smile and a question, or sharing a story of vulnerability where you stuffed up.

Trust boosts resilience

Data from the European Social Survey has shown how living in a high-trust environment increases our ability to cope in difficult times and increases resilience when dealing with discrimination, ill health or low job security.

Start by trusting yourself

Expecting others to trust you when you don't trust yourself doesn't work. Period. The late Nobel Poet Laureate Maya Angelou related, 'There is an African saying which is: Be careful when a naked person offers you a shirt. I don't trust people who don't love themselves and tell me, "I love you" '.

Trusting yourself looks like this:

- **Be okay with who you are.** Self-acceptance is about feeling at peace with yourself, including that nose, bottom or whichever body part you've fallen out of love with — your jiggly bits of imperfection. Which means replacing a critical 'Gosh, do my legs really wobble that much when I run?' with a grateful 'I feel so much better in myself for having taken up running'.

- **Give yourself permission to fail and succeed.** This is about accepting you will make mistakes. Repeatedly. Though not intentionally. This will help reduce self-criticism and being critical of others when they make mistakes. Rather than dwelling on that one critical comment in your performance review as proof positive of your failure as a person, cut yourself some slack and look at how you can use that feedback to help improve next time, and give yourself a pat on the back for all the good things that were said.

- **Believe in your own capabilities and develop an expectation of success.** If fear of failure is holding you back, what if you flipped that fear into having the courage to step forward and build on your existing strengths? It's time to trust yourself. Pushing the boundaries enables you to grow personally and professionally and increases your self-confidence.

Nurture trust in others

Your eyes meet, you're greeted with a warm smile and a firm handshake. Levels of oxytocin increase when you're in the presence of someone you like and who you're pretty sure likes you. It's released by the bucketload when we're with those we love and when a mother gives birth. Let's face it, without oxytocin it would be much harder to form a relationship with that funny-looking pink squawking bundle of joy. Its absence would be very bad news indeed for the infant, who is born so vulnerable, with no means to take care of itself.

You'll be happy to know that oxytocin is now available in a convenient nasal spray, so if you're looking for a new relationship you could do worse than head down to your local chemist and see what happens on your next Tinder date. Although a better way to boost those oxytocin levels might be to turn up as 'you', along with your best smile and a genuine interest in the other person. And to demonstrate your trustworthiness.

 We build trust through our observable trustworthy behaviour.

Should we trust our gut?

Trust has to be earned, but we instinctively know when meeting someone for the first time whether or not they are going to be trustworthy. Mostly we get it right, but on rare occasions we may fall foul of a con artist or skilled manipulator.

If when meeting someone for the first time, despite all the positive social indicators — eye contact, warm smile, firm handshake — you're left feeling something's not quite right, this uncertainty warrants follow-up.

Whatever the circumstance, when meeting someone for the first time all your brain is interested in is determining whether you're in a place of safety or danger. As noted in part I, your safety is your brain's number one priority. 'Friend or foe? Should I stay or should I go?' It determines the answer to the question in 200 milliseconds and establishes the matter of trust in just a few seconds of conversation.

But what about when you're not given the option to choose for yourself?

'Hi Belinda, this is your new teammate [or] work colleague [or] business associate.'

In this situation it's important to look for opportunities to get to know the other person quickly and work out ways to build mutual trust and respect. Note the tone and language used, the nonverbal communication of posture and gesture, and seek out those invisible threads of commonality to discover, *Hey, this person is really like me after all!*

That moment when you 'click' with someone, when your brains are in neural synchrony — it's a beautiful thing. It's why, whether you're with someone you know or someone you've only just met, you ask questions to find out what you have in common. 'And what is it you do?' being an overused starting point.

The eyes have it

In many cultures eye contact is the first step towards human connection. Someone who doesn't look you in the eye may seem shifty and untrustworthy and leave you feeling rejected. If someone is avoiding eye contact, perhaps they don't want to engage with you. You have probably done this yourself, for example to avoid being caught up by someone wanting to sell you something you don't want in the shopping mall.

Eye contact avoidance could also indicate a person is naturally shy, or that staring is culturally inappropriate — a vital consideration in our multicultural world.

How long should you look at someone? If someone stares at you for more than a few seconds it can start to make you feel uncomfortable and self-conscious. The intensity of that stare interferes with your working memory, reducing your ability to suppress irrelevant information and your imagination.

Eye contact for around three seconds feels perfect. Closer to nine or ten seconds, and it starts to get creepy!

Forging trust with touch

Trust me, I'm a doctor!

Why do we say that? Doctors and other health professionals are often highly trusted. One reason for this concerns our sense of touch. Human skin is loaded with what are called Pacinian corpuscles, which allow us to interpret the emotion being communicated. Studies have shown how *just one second of touch is sufficient to register the emotional intent of the other person.* Touch activates the orbitofrontal cortex, the part of the brain associated with reward and compassion, and activates the vagus nerve, triggering the release of oxytocin.

Touch can also have a profound effect on your ability to recover from pain and illness by helping you to relax and feel safe. That's why massage therapy is so effective in relieving muscular tension and increasing your sense of calm and wellbeing.

Psychologist Professor Dacher Keltner warns that we are now living in touch-deprived cultures, pointing to data showing that premature babies who experience human touch gain up to 47 per cent more weight than those not touched, that touch has been shown to help alleviate depression in those living with Alzheimer's, and that it doubles the likelihood of a child being willing to speak up in class.

Michelangelo said, 'to touch is to give life'. How do you use touch in your social interactions?

A 'pat on the back' indicates we've done something good. A high-five, handshake or nose rub are just a few of the physical ways we connect socially. One form of touch guaranteed to propel your oxytocin levels into outer orbit is a shared hug.

The etiquette of hugs

Hugs can be a social minefield if not used appropriately. Fortunately, a couple of simple rules of hugging etiquette can keep everyone safe.

1. **Understand the purpose of the hug.** Is this a simple meet-and-greet or is its purpose more specific, such as comforting someone who is grieving or upset?

2. **Check the person you're about to hug is okay with this.** Not everyone is into hugs or physical contact. If in doubt, the quick question 'Can I give you a hug?' is the safest approach.

Note that men and women hug differently; check it out next time you're out with friends and observe the subtle difference. Women are often more comfortable with hugging and will frequently initiate a hug with arms outstretched, clearly indicating, 'I'm coming in for the hug now'.

Men might prefer a handshake or the one-armed hug with the clasped hands held in front of the chest and body contact limited to the shoulders and chest.

In this age of raised concerns about sexual harassment it's important to understand what contact is deemed acceptable and to abide by those cultural rules. A handshake or high-five with eye contact and a warm smile will still provide the oxytocin surge desired.

How many and how long?

Paul Zak, author of *Trust Factor*, recommends eight hugs a day for greater happiness and better relationships. If you live on your own, you could always start with your cat. Though some cats can be scratchy ... a dog might be safer.

Psychotherapist Virginia Satir believes we need:

* four hugs a day for survival

* eight hugs a day for maintenance

* twelve hugs a day for growth.

Being a better giver and receiver of hugs is a great way to alleviate stress. How many hugs are you giving or receiving?

Depending on your level of comfort around being hugged, who the person hugging you is and the situation, a full-body hug can last anywhere from three to 20 seconds. This will top up your oxytocin tank wonderfully. If the prospect of 20 seconds makes you feel uncomfortable, that's okay, make it a short hug. Do what feels comfortable, whether you're into hugging trees, your kids or yourself. But if hugging isn't your thing, that's fine too.

When trust is lost

As Brené Brown reminds us, we build trust in small increments. She equates it to adding marbles to a jar. When breaches of trust occur — an unkind comment, a snide remark — marbles are taken out. Because the jar is clear glass, we can easily see how full our jar of trust is and whether it needs a little top-up. If the jar gets knocked over and all the marbles have rolled out, the question to ask is, is this jar worth refilling?

It's sad but the reality is we've probably all experienced fallouts with people we once considered good friends. You can spend years nurturing a friendship, then one ill-judged comment or argument can see that entire, fragile, carefully constructed tower of trust come tumbling down. As happened to a couple of school friends of mine.

Case Study

Mel and Gina had been besties since high school. They socialised a lot together, their families went on holiday together, and they regularly celebrated each other's successes in life and work.

Then one day Mel heard from a mutual friend about a new business Gina had set up, and that the launch party was in two weeks' time. Was Mel going to be there? Thinking this was a bit odd, but caught up interstate on business, Mel thought Gina had just forgotten to send her the invite. Strange, though, that she

---

hadn't mentioned anything about her new business venture at their last catch-up together a month or so ago.

Not sharing significant news might not have been enough to tumble the friendship, but what came next did. A phone call from another mutual friend just back from lunch with Gina and some of their other pals relaying how Gina had used the occasion to share some incredibly funny and highly embarrassing stories about Mel from a couple of years back. How everyone had laughed! Asked the friend, 'Were all those stories true?'

Mortified, Mel knew Gina had deliberately chosen to break their bond of trust. Their relationship shattered beyond redemption, they never spoke to each other again.

There is no right or wrong when it comes to relationship breakdown. The loss of trust is inevitably painful. It's also time for some serious reflection. Do you believe the relationship is salvageable, or is it time to call it quits and sever all ties? Sometimes you'll decide the relationship is worth fighting for, sometimes not.

The need for greater trust at work

Trust is critical to every interpersonal interaction in life and work. Because we invest so much time and energy into the place we call work, feeling safe to show up, to do the work you know you're capable of, to feel valued, accepted and recognised for your efforts — all these are vital.

Trusting that work is a safe environment goes way beyond physical safety. It's also about psychological safety. Harvard Business School researcher Amy Edmondson defined this as when working in a team 'you are confident that no one on the team will embarrass or punish anyone else for admitting a mistake, asking a question or offering a new idea'.

Case Study

Our friend Ben had exceptional accountancy skills, so when he was headhunted to become the CFO of a small UK-based company, he knew he would be able to contribute usefully to the organisation. His boss was technically brilliant, and Ben could see the massive potential in the range of products being developed for the health care sector that could revolutionise how certain treatments were delivered to patients.

There was only one fly in the ointment, which turned out to be the boss.

The man had absolutely no people skills and appeared to take pleasure in ridiculing his staff and being socially awkward with clients. His mood swings and inconsistent behaviour kept everyone on tenterhooks. Ben never knew whether on any given day he was going be lauded or admonished, regardless of how much effort he put into his work, which he knew to be of a very high standard. After 12 months of being fed a mixture of distortions and downright lies, Ben had had enough, because he recognised it was impacting his own wellbeing and happiness. He was conflicted because he loved the work, but he could no longer stomach working for someone who didn't share his values, whom he didn't trust and who he felt didn't trust him. With a heavy heart he handed in his resignation.

Who would you rather work for? Someone like Ben's boss with great ideas and the potential to do good but who you wouldn't trust with your own lunchbox? Or someone who was less technically talented but with their heart in the right place and the ability to draw in people who shared their vision and was aligned with their values?

Of course it would be nice to work for someone with both the technical ability and the social skills. But as Simon Sinek, author of *Start with Why*, observes, many would choose to work with someone with higher social skills that engender trust even if they lacked exceptional technical skills.

Building community

Still carried out in Amish communities in the US, a barn raising is a traditional collective activity during which a community come together to build or raise a barn for a community member. It requires careful planning, with everyone involved knowing their precise role, where they fitted in the grander scheme of things and committed to the cause.

Working (or living) alongside other people requires an understanding of difference and what works — that is, trust and strong social support to enable everyone to get on well with each other. Boosting your social network begins with the desire to be part of a 'barn-raising team'. Here you're operating in a space that feels safe but it also creates an environment where you know it's okay to disagree and challenge 'the usual' because you've got an idea for what might work better.

When you're working towards a common goal, it's easier to have those robust discussions around a point of difference, engaging in useful dialogue to negotiate agreement rather than going off in a huff if things don't go your way. Rather than seeing your colleagues as 'those idiots' who don't agree with your uniquely persuasive idea, you're open to the idea that there may be a number of perspectives to consider.

Raising social awareness in every interaction makes it easier to keep everyone around the negotiating table because trust keeps negative emotion at bay, facilitating outside-the-box thinking. Failure is no longer a disaster because your support team accepts failure as showing that you've tried, that it just didn't work out this time.

Boosting trust and connectivity at work starts with sharing — whether of ideas, your pencil sharpener or maybe a coffee — which also leads to greater mutual respect.

Elevating mutual respect

Building trust and happiness in our lives and work is also about mutual respect.

Being shown respect is about being recognised, not just as a number or a face, but as the person you are and for your capabilities, which is what Ben was seeking. At work, enjoying a high level of trust and respect makes you a more effective team member. At home, mutual respect makes you want to put in the extra effort to be a strong and loving friend, family member or partner.

Feeling recognised and acknowledged creates trust, loyalty and an understanding of how your contribution is leading towards something bigger than yourself, creating a higher sense of fulfilment and achievement.

Mutual respect starts by acknowledging we are all unique individuals with our own perspective on how the world works.

* Do you treat everyone with the same level of courtesy, consideration and kindness?

* Are you willing to listen to someone else's point of view without immediately jumping to judgement?

* Are you open to hearing someone's great new idea, even if you're not convinced it's going to go anywhere?

* Do you ensure everyone gets a chance to be heard in meetings?

* Do you encourage debate and discourse around subjects that are challenging and hard, such as how to remove the stigma around mental illness at work, or how to be more open to change and less risk averse?

* Do you listen more than you speak? (Always a toughie if you've got a lot to say.)

- Do you treat everyone in your team fairly, driving inclusivity and avoiding favouritism?

- Do you call out the good things you see being done by others? Have you recently, personally and publicly acknowledged a colleague for achieving a great outcome for the team? Have you recently sent a handwritten note of thanks or posted up the team wins in a public place where everyone gets to share in the celebration?

Often it's the smallest of gestures that have the biggest effect, like knowing the names of all your colleagues and seeking out ways to be kind.

 Our need for respect should not be underestimated.

Sadly, we commonly think about respect only when it's gone AWOL. Feeling disrespected generates a strong threat response and can seriously damage relationships. Respect matters, because as organisational psychologist Robert A. Snyder reminds us, our self-image is a lens through which we perceive all our social needs and determines our behaviour. We care deeply about what others think about us, even when we pretend we don't.

Generating mutual respect begins with:

Acknowledging the presence of another person

When you're tired at the end of a long day, and all you want to do is pop your headphones on and listen to your favourite music, but your partner desperately wants to get your attention to talk about something that's bothering them, do you:

- pretend you can't hear them

- suggest they come back in 15 minutes

- take off your headphones, look at your partner and ask, 'What's up?'

If you're busy working and a colleague pops her head around the office door or over the top of your cubicle to ask a question, do you:

* ignore her and carry on working — *can't she see you're busy?*

* tell her to go away — *make an appointment; my time is more valuable than yours*

* stop what you're doing, make eye contact and ask, 'How can I help?' or 'I'm in the middle of something right now, can I get back to you in 15?'

Acknowledgement takes only a moment, so why not choose to stop what you're doing, close the laptop, switch off the music, turn and focus on the person speaking to you.

Knowing the other person's name

If you genuinely can't remember (it's okay, most of us are terrible with names), ask them to remind you, then use it correctly. It's far better than guessing and getting it wrong — *Jeepers I've been here for six months and he STILL can't get my name right!*

Checking in on the correct pronunciation

It's not just newsreaders who need help with tricky or unusual names. If you ask the person directly how to say their name or how they like to be addressed (maybe they've got a nickname), it shows you're interested in them as a person.

Being genuinely interested in what the other person is trying to tell you

Active listening begins with eye contact (when culturally appropriate), nodding and listening before jumping in to return serve. Taking turns to speak and giving everyone equal air time, especially if the other person is naturally introverted or shy, quickly builds trust and respect.

Life is messy and relationships complex. Nurturing trust through kindness, respect and the occasional dollop of forgiveness can help keep us on track to enjoy the many splendours friendship and strong interpersonal relationships provide.

Your prescription for nurturing trust and respect

- Treat everyone with mutual respect. At home, never take your partner for granted. Check with your friends and colleagues to learn, understand and remember their individual preferences, and factor these in for better communication and collaboration. Remembering that your friend Tony is allergic to prawns will be appreciated when you ask him round for a seafood dinner!

- Stay curious about what you can improve on in your interactions with others. Do you show your appreciation for the help you receive, smile and say thank you?

- Be willing to listen to other people's ideas and points of view, whether you agree with them or not. Healthy differences allow for more robust and honest debate around issues that might affect your relationships at a personal or professional level.

- Create the time needed to build relationships.

- Take turns to speak and practise active listening. This demonstrates respect and builds trust. Feeling heard is vital to reducing fears and anxiety.

- Look for small ways to be more social, like saying hello and engaging in eye contact (when culturally appropriate) and asking questions about the other person.

- Nurture trust by being reliable, dependable, honest and fair in all your dealings. Be real! It's okay not to have all the answers, and revealing your vulnerability by asking for help is the fastest way to engender trust. People love to help!

(continued)

- Admit when you're wrong and take responsibility for your mistakes. We all stuff up from time to time.

- Seek to make connections beyond your immediate work circle. It's good to have friends across the organisation and beyond its borders.

- Join a networking group, not as an exercise for collecting business cards, but as a way to connect and build meaningful new relationships.

- At work, create what Simon Sinek calls a circle of safety where effectiveness rather than efficiency is rewarded, focusing on elevating engagement, learning opportunities and higher performance.

- Look for ways to demonstrate your trustworthiness by being consistent in how you interact with other people. Be seen as a fair player who seeks to enhance and bring out the best in others.

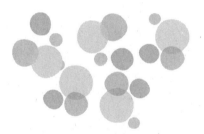

16
Kindness and compassion

Wherever there is a human being, there is an opportunity for a kindness.
Lucius Annaeus Seneca

In the dizzy excitement of our first morning in New York, we headed out from our hotel towards Central Park, weaving through the melee of busy commuters, coffees in hand. It seemed like everyone was in a rush. Were they all late, I wondered, or was this simply a reflection of the pace of life in the Big Apple?

To our horror we noticed a man lying, unmoving, in the gutter while the people streamed around him, some stepping, almost tripping, over his body as if he wasn't there. Paramedics arrived and started to assess the situation. As we moved away, I was left wondering:

When did we stop being kind?

When did we cease to register when a fellow human being was in trouble and stop to offer help?

Is our self-absorption, busyness and sense of time poverty, the urgency we feel to get to the next appointment/lunch date/tennis practice so overwhelming that we choose to turn a blind eye?

 Kindness. It costs us nothing but is invaluable for us all.

Do you consciously seek to be kind?

In the early 1970s a couple of behavioural scientists set out to explore what motivates kindness through an experiment involving Princeton theology students. In what became known as the Good Samaritan Study, some groups of students were instructed to prepare a short talk on the parable of the Good Samaritan, which they were then asked to deliver in a building nearby.

- One group was told they had plenty of time for the walk across the campus.
- Another group was assured that if they left right away, they would arrive in time.
- While another group were warned they were already running late so they should hurry over straight away.

On their way, each student encountered a person (an actor) lying on the ground in obvious distress.

Among the results, only 10 per cent of those who believed they were already late stopped to offer help, whereas 63 per cent of those who didn't feel the same time pressure stopped. Clearly for most of the former group the fear of being late for their appointment overrode any compassion they might have felt.

Would you have stopped to help? If not, what do you think would have been your reason?

Are you missing out on opportunities to show greater kindness?

We walk past homeless people on the street every day. We avoid volunteer charity workers keen to sign us up to donate to one worthy cause or another. We ignore the sound of a colleague sobbing behind the closed bathroom door.

It's about seeing the need and choosing whether or not to act on it.

When we're under time pressure and feeling stressed it's easy to get caught up in our thoughts and concerns and to stop noticing what's happening around us. But time isn't always the issue. Consumed by our own priorities we look but fail to see.

 What difference could it make to the world if we all chose to be just 5 per cent kinder?

Why kindness makes us happy

Being kind to others benefits *us*, and it's more than the hope or expectation of reciprocity.

That warm inner glow of kindness comes from activating that part of your brain associated with generosity and cooperation, the striatum.

A selfless act of kindness has been shown to increase our positive emotions. Why not set yourself the challenge of offering one small act of kindness every day for 30 days, and see what impact that has on your mood, happiness and wellbeing?

Being kind doesn't have to involve anything huge. It could be no more than:

* sharing your umbrella with someone waiting to cross the road when it's pouring with rain

* giving a stranger money for the parking meter if you notice they are struggling to find the right coins

* offering to help someone struggling with a giant suitcase up a long staircase in the metro.

But your small random act of kindness will have a significant impact on how the recipient feels for the rest of the day — happier, more trusting, and more generous in their turn, because kindness is contagious. Buying a colleague a cup of coffee gives them the idea of doing the same for someone else. It's a great example of paying it forward.

One study showed how being kind to others as well as to yourself, and actively observing kindness happening around us, boosts subjective happiness. Just a week of performing or observing one kind act a day is enough to make you feel happier. Whether you're helping a friend, a family member or a perfect stranger, the greater the number of kind acts, the greater the happiness effect.

So next time you notice your friend's got spinach stuck between their teeth, or a harassed parent valiantly trying to deal with their two-year-old's tantrum in the supermarket, or a colleague looking as if they are bearing the weight of the world on their shoulders, remember that your kindness in the moment could make all the difference.

How will you choose to be more kind? You don't have to donate a kidney (unless of course they happen to need one), but kindness makes us more prosocial, gracious and happy, which has to be good for us and the planet too.

Kindness makes us better humans

I was running late for an early-morning meeting and uncertain about the parking arrangements at the venue, which just happened to be a cathedral. As I parked in the eerily empty space (where was everyone?), I noticed a security guard approaching. *Uh-oh*, I thought, *I'm about to get told to move on.*

Instead I was greeted with a warm smile and a question about the car – we own a vintage convertible. He then proceeded to tell me about his own car, also a vintage, parked downstairs in the underground car park. Aha! So that's where I was supposed to be. Conscious of the time but not wishing to appear rude, I chatted for another minute or two before asking him for directions to the meeting room.

On my return an hour or so later to my still rather lonely vehicle I noticed a piece of paper in a plastic cover under the windscreen wipers. *Bother,* I thought, *a parking ticket.* But when I looked closer I saw it was a flyer with an invitation to attend a church service and on the back, handwritten, four words: 'Permission to park OK' and the signature of the security guard.

Compassion protects our physical and mental wellbeing

Kindness is the product of compassion and, suggests Emiliana Simon-Thomas of the Greater Good Science Center at Berkeley, the key to our wellbeing, because 'no matter who we are, when things get difficult, we benefit from social support'. She explains how 'experiences of compassion involve several processes that together make us feel more connected to others, more personally effective, more intrinsically motivated and inclined to be generous — all factors that drive engagement, innovation and performance'.

Compassion is believed to protect our wellbeing through its buffering effect against stress and redirection of focus to others. This prosocial effect creates stronger interpersonal connection while also strengthening the immune system, reducing inflammation and helping us to recover from illness more quickly. It can even extend our life.

Other benefits include:

+ better acceptance of adversity and ability to move past negative emotion

+ lower rates of anxiety and depression

+ lower stress through reduced cortisol levels and better emotional self-regulation

+ increased optimism, curiosity and initiative

+ stronger relationships and demonstrations of forgiveness and empathy.

What's more, it makes us more attractive as people and uplifts others around us.

Dacher Keltner from the University of California believes we share a compassionate instinct with many other animals, including rats and chimpanzees. Studies have shown how very young children will spontaneously demonstrate compassion and helpful behaviour without being taught.

The expression 'survival of the fittest' is commonly attributed to Charles Darwin, author of *On the Origin of Species*, though it was the English philosopher Herbert Spencer who coined it in his book *The Principles of Sociology*. Darwin argued that 'communities that included the greatest number of sympathetic members would flourish best and rear the greatest number of offspring'. This idea came to be referred to as the 'survival of the kindest'.

If you've ever leaned back uneasily in the dentist's chair before a major procedure, or worried about how well you're going to fit into your new role, or waited anxiously for those test results that won't be ready until Monday next week, you'll probably remember how much better you felt after a few words of reassurance, of feeling connected to as a person. This is not just your imagination. Having reviewing 250 scientific papers for their book *Compassionomics: The Revolutionary Scientific Evidence that Caring Makes a Difference*, doctors Stephen Trzeciak and Anthony Mazzarelli found that taking time to show compassion has measurable benefits for both doctors and patients.

And it's true for all our relationships. Caring about others and feeling cared for is what makes the difference. Caring is one of the greatest gifts we can share to reduce stress and the risk of burnout.

Cultivating kindness and compassion

Compassion inspires us to be kind. It is the core component of love, sympathy and empathy. It helps us to show we care and brings us together as humans. When compassion is absent, something very powerful is lost, which is why seeking to live a life of kindness and compassion matters.

Compassion for others starts with having compassion for ourselves

'If you don't love yourself,' the Dalai Lama is said to have remarked, 'you cannot love others …. If you have no compassion for yourself then you are not capable of developing compassion for others. I believe compassion to be one of the few things we can practice that will bring immediate and long-term happiness to our lives'.

If you're forever beating yourself up for making a mistake, for saying the wrong thing or for not getting the result you hoped for, please stop. Your self-inflicted wounds, while painful and slow to heal, are also damaging. It's time to cast off the sackcloth and ashes and start practising self-acceptance.

Researcher and Associate Professor Kristen Neff describes self-compassion as kindness to ourselves that is gentle, supportive and understanding, and it sets the standard for how we respond to others.

Self-compassion is about treating yourself as though you were responding to the suffering of a good friend. If you're not sure what this might look like, ask yourself, *How would I respond to someone I could see was hurting? What words would I use? What actions might I take?*

Forgive yourself

Forgiving ourselves our daily trespasses is about tuning in to the story you're telling yourself, checking: Is this the truth or just my version of events? What narrative is your inner critic sharing that needs to be challenged or better understood? The desire to fit in, to be deemed worthy of belonging, can lead us to adopt a mindset of creating impossible standards for ourselves that set us up to fail. Give yourself permission to be imperfect and to make mistakes.

Know you are not alone

We *all* make mistakes. We are all fallible and vulnerable. We feel the same pain and emotions as others experiencing the same trauma, so rather than choosing to withdraw or socially isolate ourselves we can stay strong knowing we are not alone in our struggles.

Identify what you want and practise self-compassion as you set about achieving your goals. If perfectionism or impostordom are getting in your way, how can you loosen those shackles of self-criticism by changing your internal dialogue to be less judgemental?

Practise mindful self-compassion meditation

There are many excellent resources in this space. If you are new to the practice, I recommend visiting Kristin Neff's website where you'll find a number of guided meditations to get you started and a questionnaire to test your current level of self-compassion.

 Kindness and compassion strengthen connection.

Your prescription for greater kindness and compassion

- **Take the challenge!** Choose to undertake an act of kindness every day. Big or small, for yourself or another person, ramp up your happy vibes.

- **Start with a smile.** Emotions are contagious. Connecting with others is as simple as sharing positive emotion with a smile and cheery hello.

- **Take action to put things right.** This is compassion at work. You've seen that someone needs help. Your compassion is in the actions you take to help them out.

- **Focus outwards.** Remembering a colleague's birthday, shouting a friend a coffee or buying a thoughtful birthday gift demonstrates you care, strengthening relationships, boosting mood and elevating happiness.

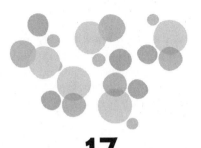

17

Empathy: 'I feel your pain'

Nobody cares how much you know,
until they know how much you care.
Theodore Roosevelt

Empathy means identifying with someone who is doing it tough. Your heightened sensitivity and understanding means you can imagine and feel their pain. Forging deeper social connections helps us to better understand our own emotions.

We all make mistakes. An empathetic response helps to give you the courage and confidence to find a solution and make things right. Those small words of encouragement that demonstrate genuine care and understanding inspire you to change.

Without empathy it's hard to be sure what another person might be thinking or feeling. This uncertainty can result in our jumping to conclusions or making false assumptions because we haven't taken the time to tap into 'what's really going on here'.

Case Study

Penny was in her early forties, happily married with two gorgeous kids. She was one of those people who always had a smile on her face, her glass always half full. She had a good job in a company that clearly recognised her talents. All was well in her world – until she started getting bad headaches.

At first, she said, they happened only a couple of times a month, but their frequency, intensity and duration were increasing. A scan was arranged, and the presence of her brain tumour couldn't be denied. Worse still, it was aggressive and had already shown signs of metastasis.

There is no good way to tell someone they are going to die.

She was referred to a highly respected surgeon and an oncologist, both of whom were kind and compassionate and did what they could. But while she continued to put on a brave face, Penny was angry, sad and scared. Frightened about what lay ahead, and worried how her husband and children would cope once she was gone.

While I could do nothing to change the harsh reality, I could act as a sounding board. We had many long chats. We talked, laughed and cried together, but for much of the time I just listened. She spoke at length about her fears, how angry she was at being short-changed by life and her hopes for the future of her kids. Her courage and deep love for her family helped to prepare them, and her, for her last journey.

The hardest part of being a doctor is having to tell someone they have a terminal illness and their time is limited.

 We all seek to be heard and understood.

When out for dinner with your nearest and dearest, the one thing that can make or break your evening isn't the food or the ambience of the restaurant; it's the care and attention — that is, the level of interest—shown you by your waitperson. The one thing that will keep you at your job isn't access to a gym or great coffee; it's feeling consistently acknowledged as a person and asked, 'How are things going?'

How has empathy shown up in your life?

The brainy facts about empathy

If you've ever winced when you've seen someone slam their hand in the car door or bump their head on a low door frame, or felt your heart race as you watch Olympic sprinters fly towards the finish line, your response is due to what are known as mirror neurons.

These were first identified by Giacomo Rizzolatti and his team from the University of Parma in their work on macaque monkeys. They were able to show how neurons in a monkey's brain would light up both when undertaking an action such as picking up a peanut or when watching another monkey doing the same thing. This led to the hypothesis that this was the physiological basis of empathy, the process by which we identify intuitively with another person.

Empathy aligns us or puts us 'in sync' with another person. When we're out of sync it's more difficult to feel connected and understanding. Perhaps you've noticed this yourself.

In her book *The Empathy Effect* psychiatrist Helen Riess describes the three components of empathy:

1. emotional resonance, courtesy of your mirror neurons

2. cognition to understand that the pain is unique to the sufferer and to be able to hold your own perspective of their situation

3. concern to respond and take care of the other person.

The benefits of empathy

Empathy provides a means of building social connection. Understanding why your friend is so upset about losing their pet, or appreciating what thoughts might be going through your boss's mind knowing the company is experiencing a major downturn, makes it easier to respond appropriately and compassionately.

Empathy helps us to help others. That's why friends rally round to bring cooked meals, offer to baby-sit or take us out for coffee when they know we're in a difficult space.

 Showing empathy towards others helps us better manage our own emotions during times of stress.

Empathy makes a real difference to how you feel about your work. Working for an empathetic boss will alleviate your stress and increase your confidence and capability, while at the same time reducing your boss's risk of mood disorder, burnout and heart attack. Win–win! Demonstrating empathy boosts your awareness of your own emotional needs while reducing stress and your risk of burnout.

Patients in the care of empathetic doctors rate their surgeons as more caring, rate their surgical outcomes twenty times more highly and enjoy quicker recovery.

Empathy is linked to higher job satisfaction. Which is why in the corporate world the manager who genuinely cares about their employees, is interested in their health and wellbeing, and is willing to provide the support and resources needed for everyone to do their work well, is the boss we all want to work for.

The 2019 State of Workplace Empathy Study from Businesssolver reported that 93 per cent of employees said they were more likely to stay with an empathetic leader and 92 per cent of CEOs believed their organisation to be empathetic. Not only that, 82 per cent of employees said they would change jobs to work with a more empathetic leader and 78 per cent said they would work harder for an empathetic leader.

So let me ask you a question. Would you prefer to work for a company where:

a.   profits come before people, but you receive a fabulous salary

b.   you are paid less but treated as an individual and encouraged to grow professionally and personally?

 Demonstrating empathy is a skill that can be learned or enhanced.

Empathy precedes compassion, which is the conscious, sympathetic awareness of another person's misfortune accompanied by a desire to alleviate it. Let's take a look at what helps kindle the empath within.

Building empathy

We are all born with the capacity for empathy but it is also a skill set that can be learned and developed.

Look up

Engaging in eye contact shows the other person you're ready to interact. If you've ever heard yourself say impatiently, 'Look at me when I'm talking to you!' you'll know how it feels when you're trying to say something important but are struggling to get the other person's attention. Saying hello and meeting someone's gaze tells them, 'I see you'.

Listen

Active listening means paying close attention to what your colleague is saying. Showing you're listening can involve stopping what else you are doing (closing your laptop, turning off your mobile phone), watching for non-verbal cues, leaning in towards the other person, nodding and perhaps even paraphrasing them to confirm you understand them.

Are you really listening, or just going through the motions?

Stay curious

Whether you're sitting on a bus, catching a taxi or standing in line at the check-in desk at the airport there are myriad opportunities to engage a stranger in conversation. It's much more than just passing the time of day, or being nosey — it's a golden opportunity to get curious about what's going on in another person's head and engage with different viewpoints and perspectives.

Dr Martin Seligman, founder of Positive Psychology, sees curiosity as a key way to improve life satisfaction. Children are always inquisitive, and they're not afraid to ask questions, so why should you be afraid to extend your social circle?

Choose not to judge

Judgemental? Who, me?

We pass judgement all the time. We're very good at it and, yes, sometimes enjoy it.

'Did you see those shoes — what was she thinking?'

'No shirt, scruffy hair, clearly hasn't taken a shower in a while — what a loser!'

'I wouldn't trust him — his eyes are too close together.'

Challenging those thoughts with an empathic approach requires parking all that judgement (tricky if all the judgement parking bays in your head are already full), sitting with the whole person in front of you and staying curious about who they are. Showing empathy towards someone who doesn't share your beliefs will elevate your skill to a new level, but is incredibly important for those times when you have to work alongside or interact with people you think of as very different from you. Bringing empathy to all your interactions will strengthen the relationship on both sides.

Watch the tone

Identifying the emotion someone is experiencing includes paying attention to their tone of voice. This will help you to judge how to interact and respond.

At my dad's funeral, feeling intensely sad, my voice cracked as I struggled to deliver the eulogy. After the service, while mingling with family members and friends, I couldn't help but notice the general tone of reciprocal kindness and compassion in the gentle exchanges.

Empathy can help save the day when dealing with righteous indignation too. It's natural to get upset when external factors add an extra layer of complexity or challenge to your day. One time an international flight I was on was delayed interminably. We'd been kept waiting sitting on the tarmac for over three hours without explanation, and rising levels of vexation were leading to loud and angry exchanges between passengers and staff. As much in the dark as everyone else, the cabin crew struggled valiantly to defuse the tense situation by adopting an empathetic approach. They were able to settle many fraying tempers by listening to and identifying with the travellers' frustration. When the announcement finally came that we would shortly be taking off, the whole cabin erupted into cheers, applause and smiles of relief.

Stay on the level

One of the first things we were taught as medical students was to ensure we adopted an open posture and never talked down to people. 'Uncross those arms, Brockis. You're looking defensive!' Actually, I was just cold, but my closed posture could be interpreted by my patients to indicate I was authoritarian, unapproachable or aloof.

When setting up my own medical practice I took pains to ensure there was plenty of space to sit alongside my patients. Whether in an interview or chatting to a colleague in an open-plan office, you'll feel more connected when the conversation is held with both parties at the same level. That's why doctors who get down on their hands and knees when talking with a child or perch on the end of the bed when speaking with a patient are seen as more empathetic and caring.

How do you level up with people?

Empathy, says Emiliana Simon-Thomas 'is an inborn reflex for understanding all emotions that we can strengthen or suppress. When strengthened we are more socially adept and appealing, we're better on teams and leading. Learning to channel our empathy into compassion for another person's suffering serves to quieten our own inner self-critic ...'.

Being empathetic will ensure you are more adaptive to change, keep you safe and make you a kinder person.

Your prescription for elevating empathy

- **Be interested in people.** Seek to understand what others may be experiencing.

- **Keep your own stress in check.** That way you remain receptive and open to what's going on around you.

- **Switch off your technological devices.** Engage in real-time, face-to-face conversation.

- **Get enough sleep.** It's hard to be empathetic when you're tired beyond caring.

- **Check your internal language.** If judgement is getting in the way, try curiosity instead.

- **Express gratitude.** This enhances compassion and boosts empathy by attuning you to the actions and perspectives of others.

Conclusion:
The times are
a-changin',
and so can you

*The greatest discovery of my generation is that a human being
can alter his life by altering his attitudes.*
William James

Well done for making it this far. Whatever your reason for picking
up this book, by now I hope you have a better understanding of
the wealth of opportunities available to you to become the best
version of yourself, to successfully weather the storms of life and
to stay safe as you adapt and thrive. How you can bring about
the change you desire — whether it's to feel happier, healthier or
more connected — will come down to three things:

- **knowing** what it takes to create greater happiness for
  your emotional and mental wellbeing

- **choosing** those aspects of your lifestyle and environment that best enable you to thrive

- **seeking** ways to stay connected at the human level.

Small changes

True life is lived when tiny changes occur.
Leo Tolstoy

If you've consciously and successfully introduced a positive change in your life in the past, you'll know how tweaking an existing habit or making one small change can create a ripple effect. Perhaps you've seen it demonstrated by a friend or colleague: they began with the intention of abstaining from alcohol for a month, say, which led to healthier eating choices, which in turn encouraged them to start an exercise program.

As soon as you see or feel the positives that good change can bring, you get the bonus of the reward (remember those dopamine cupcakes?). Anticipating the reward works as a powerful motivator, encouraging you to make further improvements, as my colleague Kylie discovered.

Taking on that first modest goal had led Kylie to embrace a whole raft of other positive changes without much additional effort. Rather than thinking you've got to commit to a radical package of new practices, sometimes the smallest of tweaks to your mindset and behaviour will produce the greatest positive impact.

Perhaps you've already had this experience. If not, but you're eager to make it happen now, let's look at how best to prepare for the challenge of successful goal achievement or, as Mahatma Gandhi put it, of 'being the change we wish to see'.

Case Study

At our first meeting, my impression of Kylie was of a super-smart, ambitious young woman, passionate about her work and very good at it. She was already operating in a senior managerial role and had some big hairy audacious goals for where she wanted to be in five years' time. She was on a mission.

Working very long hours, she was also highly stressed and frustrated by the less than stellar work behaviours of some of her colleagues. With wedding plans on the horizon, she never had the time to exercise and was carrying extra kilos, which made her feel depressed.

Then along came an opportunity to participate in a work-based fundraiser. This required everyone in the office to commit to rowing a set number of kilometres every day on a stationary rowing machine.

Never one to shy away from a challenge, she got stuck in and was soon spending an hour on the rower five days a week. As she rowed herself to greater fitness, her desire for more exercise grew and she began going to the gym regularly.

Not surprisingly, the kilos started melting away, and as her body and mood changed she started paying more attention to her diet. Feeling happier and more energised, she now had the mental space to begin tackling the performance issues at the office, and this led to a significant improvement in the workplace environment. Soon everyone was lifting their game, not just on the rowing machine, but through improved performance, collaboration, working relationships and communication.

Nine months later she had ticked all the boxes. She was happier, more energised, fitter, healthier and getting on well with all her colleagues.

Where are you now?

No, I don't mean are you reading this in bed or on your way to work. Where are you in your life? Are you:

* feeling completely stuck
* in a holding pattern, waiting for a new direction
* moving along comfortably, confidently dealing with the rough and the smooth?

Having a clear idea of where you are now, even if it's not where you want to be, is important because it provides you with a baseline from which to measure your progress.

Keep calm and move forward boldly

At home we have a mug emblazoned with the comforting words 'Keep Calm and Call Dad'. It's sound advice in times of crisis in our household, and having grown up with a super-practical Mr Fixit dad who never gets fazed by problems, our kids have frequently followed it. His eyes light up with the prospect of a challenge, and the opportunity to put together a nice Excel spreadsheet, while the rest of us are reassured that 'all will be well', because the engineer in him will never allow him to give up until a solution is found.

Even if you're not an engineer with a terrier-like tenacity for fixing things (or married to one), you can find your own inner calm by tapping into your values, understanding what really matters to you, knowing what you want and aligning your mindset to being a winner. This will provide you with the courage to step forward and embrace the change you are about to embark on.

Where to start

This is about identifying:

* what you want to be doing more of
* what behaviour needs to stop
* what you can carry on doing.

This book has covered a lot of ground. I hope it hasn't overwhelmed you (especially if overwhelm has become your middle name and is just the problem you want to fix). My aim has been to help you determine:

1. what's currently missing from your life that could increase your level of happiness, improve your wellbeing and boost your sense of belonging

2. what resources and support you need to make the change

3. what to do next.

Remember, it *all* counts. Getting better at managing your emotional and mental wellbeing and feeling happier is as important as engaging in self-care to fully thrive and nurturing strong relationships. First choose the area you think needs your most urgent attention. If you are unsure, try jotting down your three to five biggest pain points and ordering them according to the degree of pain they are causing. If it's a tie for first place, choose either one; you'll be getting onto the second item as soon as you've fixed the first.

'But Jenny, the biggest problem I have is *out of my control.*'

Aha. This matters, because you can expend an awful lot of time, energy and emotion worrying, fretting and gnashing your teeth over things that you have no influence over. Infuriating as it is — because I get that you want this fixed — this is when it's time to pull back and consider letting this one go. Because no matter how much you would love things to be different, where they are totally out of your control, the question to ask yourself is, *What is the cost to my health, happiness and wellbeing if I remain locked in this unresolvable struggle?*

The strength of your desire

If you've lots of experience in setting yourself goals, you'll know how some are easier to achieve than others, some are abandoned en route and some end up getting tossed out because you realise you've set yourself the wrong target.

What's important to determine is *the strength of your desire.*

How much do you really want this?

You might like the sound of a thriver's mindset, but is it an imperative no-matter-what or a nice-to-have, meh?

It's time to assess the strength of your desire against your commitment to making the change. Rate it on a scale of 1 to 10, where 1 is weak and 10 is a passionate ambition.

Say your desire to develop a thriver's mindset comes in at an 8. Great, you're definitely tapping into something you want. But if your commitment level is at a 3–4, uh-oh, Houston we have a problem. Unless your commitment is aligned to the strength of your desire and at a minimum of 7, success is likely to elude you.

The magic trifecta to win the day is commitment to the cause, consistency of application and persistence. Without the strong desire for and commitment to making things different, nothing will change because your deep attachment to your existing habits makes successful habit change a challenge.

Anything less than a 7 for commitment might mean one of the following:

1. **You're not ready.** There's other stuff happening that needs to be dealt with first. Best to wait.

2. **You're self-sabotaging.** What is your head telling you? That you can't, that it's not possible, that it's selfish to focus on yourself? These are typical excuses, justifications or rationalisations your mind can come up with. Side hustles can sideswipe the best of intentions. Best to deal with them first.

3. **You're kidding yourself that this matters to you.** You're actually managing the expectations of others. Oops. Time to regroup and check in what's right for YOU.

Time for action and responsibility

This is where the rubber hits the road. While not wanting to sound like your mother telling you what to do, this is where it's up to you, to take action and assume the responsibility that goes with it. You may believe you need to catch the 347 bus to your destination, but you could still be sitting at the bus stop in three weeks' time if you forgot to check the 347 is still running on that route. Oh, and you are the driver. Did I forget to share that small detail?

The driver of your change

Getting permission to proceed can be tough, especially when you're the one signing the permission slip. How often have you deferred progress to go for a walk or taken time out for a bit of 'me time' because of societal or cultural expectation?

Remember, you have the power to lead change because you're already in the driver's seat with your permission slip signed and the roadmap in front of you.

Your neurobiology makes behavioural change difficult, because your brain is hardwired to keep you safe; it's a great big prediction machine that seeks out familiar patterns. It would far rather you stayed put in the comfy armchair of the status quo. Your brain would much rather conserve your finite mental juices for those higher-order executive thoughts around organising, planning, focusing and decision making than expending time and energy forming new neural pathways that require considerable practice and upkeep.

We evolved as creatures of habit to conserve energy, and your brain will fight hard to keep to the existing pathways. After all, you may have spent years embedding the habits that got you here, even if they no longer serve you well.

Leading effective change

Many of your subconscious habits and automated behaviours, like your ability to drive a car, are enormously helpful; others, such as eating snack foods in front of the goggle box every night 'to relax' or smoking to 'calm your nerves', are less so. The more you practise your habits and rituals, the stronger and more deeply embedded your neural circuitry becomes.

Whether it's about feeling better about yourself as a person, feeling happier or more content with what you already have, finding a solution to regaining the vitality and energy you need to power through your day, or understanding your colleagues better, this is about first determining what you want.

You are way more powerful than you probably give yourself credit for. As my husband, a diehard Eddie Izzard fan, likes to quip, 'The power of the force within you is strong'.

And here's the thing: you're already probably doing a lot of what's been covered in the book, and doing well. Time for a quick pat on the back — maybe give yourself a bit of a hug (because hugging is good for us, as you know). It's always reassuring to know you're doing okay.

The evidence from the science is compelling. You can learn to successfully embed new ways of thinking and doing, to supersede those habits that no longer serve you well, using techniques shown by the research to work. Overcoming the modern maladies of high stress, overwork, mental distress and social disconnection is not only possible; you already have the capability and capacity to make it happen.

Here are a few tips to foster success:

Keep the change small

Trying to introduce a radical overhaul of your life all at once is doomed to failure. Starting low and adding one small change at a time will be far less painful and far more successful. James Clear, author of *Atomic Habits*, recommends 1 per cent improvements. That sounds manageable, doesn't it?

Augment a pre-existing habit

If you've already made an effort to say thank you more often to your friends and colleagues, augmenting your gratitude practice could look like:

- buying coffee or lunch for them
- making it public by posting a thank you online
- writing a personal note or letter of thanks.

Make it evergreen

A lousy habit that gives us no joy is destined for the habit bin. It won't work. With every new habit you consider, make it attractive, easy, satisfying (you did it!) and obvious. For example, you can see the delicious fruit you bought at the market because you arrange it in your fruit bowl, rather than storing it away in the fridge. Clear defines habits as 'the compound interest of self-improvement'.

Keep track of it

As with keeping a gratitude journal, monitoring your progress by keeping a written record of it is highly rewarding (dopamine cupcakes for you!) and motivates you to persevere. The Headspace meditation tracker does this by recording how many days in a row you've practised your meditation. This is great if, like me, you find it sparks an obsessive determination not to break the chain.

Work to a time frame

Choose a start and finish date and mark them in your calendar where they are visible.

I usually suggest allowing 90 days — long enough to establish your new habit and achieve your goal, but not so long that you get bored with your efforts. According to folklore it takes only

21 days to create the beautiful new version of you, but some researchers suggest an average of 66 days depending on the complexity of the desired new habit, the strength of your desire to achieve it, and the support you have to hold you to your word.

Find an accountability buddy

Share your goal for change with your partner, a family friend or a colleague, so they can help keep you accountable. They may even choose to accompany you on your journey. For example, buddy groups for weight loss are more effective than flying solo, and you get to celebrate your wins along the way.

Life is not perfect

You are not perfect, but you are perfectly adapted to follow the path that will enable you to:

- enjoy greater happiness by embracing your full spectrum of emotions, cherishing the positives that come from gratitude, helping others, purpose and meaning, mindfulness and adopting a thriver's mindset

- relish the energy and vitality that come from greater physical and mental wellbeing and the support crew of nature, music and dance, laughter and play

- savour your ability to form strong relationships that create deep connection and a sense of belonging based on trust, kindness, compassion and empathy.

Are you ready to be the truly happy, thriving human you know you can be?

A note from Jenny

To help you achieve your goals I've created a resources page on my website (drjennybrockis.com/resources) that provides a whole raft of tips, strategies and further information to support you on your journey.

If you want to stay in touch and keep up to date with the latest findings from the world of neuroscience and positive psychology, I write a weekly blog, host regular webinars and post articles on LinkedIn each week.

If you're interested in finding out more about how we can work together, whether through a speaking event, workshop or workplace program, let's connect.

If you've enjoyed this book and it has helped you make some positive changes to nurture your Thriving Mind, I'd love to hear your story.

Jenny

drjennybrockis.com

www.drjennybrockis.com

LinkedIn: drjennybrockis
Twitter: @drjennybrockis
Instagram: @drjennybrockis
Facebook: dr jennybrockis

References

Part I: Disruption

1. Don't panic, but dinner is burning in the oven

Pencavel, J. (2013). 'The Productivity of Working Hours', *Discussion Papers* 13–006, Stanford Institute for Economic Policy Research.

Kivimaki, M. et al. (2015). 'Long working hours and risk of coronary heart disease and stroke: A systematic review and meta-analysis of published and unpublished data for 603,838 individuals', *The Lancet*, 31 October, 1739–46.

World Health Organization (2019). 'Burn-out an "occupational phenomenon": International Classification of Diseases', *Mental Health Evidence and Research* (MER), 28 May.

Pieper, J. (1948, 1st edn). *Leisure: The Basis of Culture*, St Augustine's Press.

'About the Workaholics Anonymous 12-Step Recovery Program', recovery.org, 18 December 2019.

Pfeffer, J. (2018). *Dying for a Paycheck: How Modern Management Harms Employee Health and Company Performance — and What We Can Do About It*, HarperCollins.

Maslach, C., and Jackson, S.E. (1981). 'The measurement of experienced burnout', *Journal of Occupational Behaviour* 2, 99–113.

Schaufeli, W.B., De Witte, H., and Desart, S. (2019). Manual Burnout Assessment Tool (BAT). Unpublished internal report, KU Leuven, Belgium.

O'Reilly, J., Robinson, J.L., Berdahl, S.L., and Banki, S. (2014). 'Is Negative Attention Better Than No Attention? The Comparative Effects of Ostracism and Harassment at Work', *Organization Science* 26(3), 4 April.

Virgin Pulse (2015), 'Labour of Love: What Employees Love about Work and Ways to Keep the Spark Alive', virginpulse.com, 4 February.

Mann, A. (2018). 'Why We Need Best Friends at Work', Gallup Workplace, 15 January.

Lyubomirsky, S. (2009). *The How of Happiness: A New Approach to Getting the Life You Want*, Penguin Putnam.

AC Nielsen (2018). The Nielsen Total Audience Report Q2 2018, Media Insights, 12 December.

Murthy, V. (2017). 'Work and the Loneliness Epidemic', *Harvard Business Review.*

Australian Psychological Society and Swinburne University (2018). *The Australian Loneliness Report*, November.

Ninivaggi, F.J. (2019). 'Loneliness: A New Epidemic in the USA', *Psychology Today*, 12 February.

Jo Cox Commission on Loneliness, *Combatting Loneliness One Conversation at a Time: A Call to Action*, jocoxfoundation.org.

Holt-Lunstad, J., Smith, T.B., Baker, M., Harris, T. et al. (2015). 'Loneliness and Social Isolation as Risk Factors for Mortality: A Meta-Analytic Review', *Perspectives on Psychological Science* 10(2), 227–37.

Part II: Happiness

Achor, S. (2010). *The Happiness Advantage: The Seven Principles That Fuel Success and Performance at Work*, Virgin Books.

Waldinger, R. (2016). 'What makes a good life? Lessons from the longest study on happiness', TED talk, 25 January.

Buettner, D. (2008). *The Blue Zones: Lessons for Living Longer from the People Who've Lived the Longest*, Penguin.

Zak, P. (2017). 'The Neuroscience of Trust', *Harvard Business Review*, January–February.

Robak, R., and Griffin, P. (2012). 'Purpose in life: What is its relationship to happiness, depression, and grieving?' *North American Journal of Psychology* 2, 113–19.

3. Purpose and meaning – for a reason

Hill, P.L., and Turiano, N.A. (2014). 'Purpose in Life as a Predictor of Mortality across Adulthood', *Psychological Science* 25(7), 1482–6.

Cohen, R., Bavishi, C., and Rozanski, A. (2015). 'Purpose in Life and Its Relationship to All-Cause Mortality and Cardiovascular Events', *Psychosomatic Medicine* 1.

Turner, A.D., Smith, C.E., and Ong, J.C. (2017). 'Is purpose in life associated with less sleep disturbance in older adults?', *Sleep Science Practice* 1, 14.

Lewis, N.A., Turiano, Payne, B.R., and Hill, P.L. (2017). 'Purpose in life and cognitive functioning in adulthood', *Aging, Neuropsychology, and Cognition* 24(6), 662–71.

Fredrickson, B.L., Grewen, K.M., Coffey, K.A. et al. (2013). 'Gene expression and well-being', *Proceedings of the National Academy of Sciences* 110(33), 13684–9.

Ulrich, D., and Ulrich, W. (2010). *The Why of Work: How Great Leaders Build Abundant Organisations That Win*, McGraw-Hill.

Zukin, C., and Szeltner, M. (2012). *Talent Report: What Workers Want in 2012*. Net Impact. Rutgers University.

YouGov (2014). 'Crunch Time: Why Purpose Is Everything to the Modern Workforce', callingbrands.com.

4. Grateful for gratitude

Emmons, R.A. (2008). *Thanks! How Practising Gratitude Can Make You Happier*, Houghton Mifflin Harcourt, New York.

Emmons, R.A., and Mishra, A. (2010). *Why Gratitude Enhances Well-Being: What We Know, What We Need to Know*, Oxford University Press.

Emmons, R., and McCulloch, M. (2003). 'Counting Blessings Versus Burdens: An Experimental Investigation of Gratitude and Subjective Well-Being in Daily Life', *Journal of Personality and Social Psychology* 84(2), 377–89.

Wood, A.M., Lloyd, J.S., and Atkins, S. (2009). 'Gratitude influences sleep through the mechanism of pre-sleep cognitions', *Journal of Psychosomatic Research* 66(1), 43–8.

Mills, P.J., Chopra, D., Redwine, L. et al. (2015). 'The Role of Gratitude in Spiritual Well-Being in Asymptomatic Heart Failure Patients', *Spirituality in Clinical Practice*, published online 6 April.

Seligman, M. (2002). *Authentic Happiness: Use the New Positive Psychology to Realize Your Potential for Lasting Fulfillment*, Random House Australia.

Sharma, R.S. (1999). *The Monk Who Sold His Ferrari: A Fable about Fulfilling Your Dreams and Reaching Your Destiny*, Harper Element.

5. Helping out helps everyone

Doré, B.P., Morris, R.R., Burr, D.A. et al. (2017). 'Helping Others Regulate Emotion Predicts Increased Regulation of One's Own Emotions and Decreased Symptoms of Depression', *Personality and Social Psychology Bulletin* 43(5), 729–39.

Yeung, J.W.K., Zhang, Z, and Kim, T.Y. (2017). 'Volunteering and health benefits in general adults: Cumulative effects and forms', *BMC Public Health* 18(1), 8.

Tabassum, F., Mohan, J., and Smith, P. (2016). 'Association of volunteering with mental well-being: A lifecourse analysis of a national population-based longitudinal study in the UK', *BMJ Open* 6(8), e011327.

Jenkinson, C.E., Dickens, A.P., Jones, K. et al. (2013). 'Is volunteering a public health intervention? A systematic review and meta-analysis of the health and survival of volunteers', *BMC Public Health* 13, 773.

Santi, J. (2015). *The Giving Way to Happiness: Stories and Science Behind the Transformative Power of Giving*, Tarcher Books, Penguin Group USA.

Luks, A. (1991). *The Healing Power of Doing Good*, Fawcett Columbine.

Poulin, M.J., Brown, S.L., Dillard, A.J. et al. (2013). 'Giving to Others and the Association Between Stress and Mortality', *American Journal of Public Health* 103(9), 1649–55.

Raposa, E.B., Laws, H.B., and Ansell, E.B. (2015). 'Prosocial Behavior Mitigates the Negative Effects of Stress in Everyday Life', *Clinical Psychological Science.*

Sneed, R.S., and Cohen, S. (2013). 'A prospective study of volunteerism and hypertension risk in older adults', *Psychology and Aging* 28(2), 578–86.

Schreier, H.M.C. (2013). 'Effect of Volunteering on Risk Factors for Cardiovascular Disease in Adolescents, *JAMA Pediatrics.*

Milankovic, M. (2012). 'Effects of volunteerism and relationship status on empathy', Studies by Undergraduate Researchers at Guelph (SURG) 6(1), Fall.

Mogilner, C., and Chance, Z. 'Giving Time Gives You Time', *Psychological Science* 23(10), 1233–8.

6. Mindfully yours

Moll, J., Krueger, F., Zahn, R. et al. (2006). 'Human fronto–mesolimbic networks guide decisions about charitable donation', *Proceedings of the National Academy of Sciences* 103(42), 15623–8.

Davidson, R.J., and Lutz, A. (2008). 'Buddha's Brain: Neuroplasticity and Meditation', *IEEE Signal Processing Magazine* 25(1), 174–6.

Janssen M, Heerkens, Y, and Kuijer, W. et al. (2018). 'Effects of mindfulness-based stress reduction on employees' mental health: A systematic review', *PLoS One* 13(1), e0191332.

Kuyken, W., Warren, F.C., Taylor, R.S. et al. 'Efficacy of Mindfulness-Based Cognitive Therapy in Prevention of Depressive Relapse: An Individual Patient Data Meta-analysis from Randomized Trials', *JAMA Psychiatry* 73(6), 565–74.

McGonigal, K. (2016). *The Upside of Stress: Why Stress Is Good for You and How to Get Good at It*, Penguin.

7. Laugh and play makes your day

Federation of American Societies for Experimental Biology (2010). 'Body's response to repetitive laughter is similar to the effect of repetitive exercise, study finds', *ScienceDaily*, 26 April.

Segerstrom, S.C., and Miller, G.E. (2004). 'Psychological Stress and the Human Immune System: A Meta-Analytic Study of 30 Years of Inquiry', *Psychological Bulletin* 130(4), 601–30.

Bennett, M.P., and Lengacher, C. (2009). 'Humor and Laughter May Influence Health; IV. Humor and Immune Function', *Evidence Based Complementary and Alternative Medicine* 6(2), 159–64.

Savage, B.M., Lujan, H.L., Thipparthi, R.R. et al. (2017). 'Humor, laughter, learning, and health! A brief review', *Advances in Physiology Education* 41(3).

Miller, M., and Fry, W.F. (2009). 'The effect of mirthful laughter on the human cardiovascular system', *Medical Hypotheses* 73(5), 636–9.

Bennett, M.P., Zeller, J.M., Rosenberg, L. et al. (2003). 'The Effect of Mirthful Laughter on Stress and Natural Killer Cell Activity', *Alternative Therapies in Health and Medicine* 9(2), 38–45.

Svebak, S., Romundstad, S., and Holmen, J. 'A 7-year prospective study of sense of humor and mortality in an adult county population: The HUNT-2 study', *International Journal of Psychiatry in Medicine* 40, 125–46.

Bains, G.S., Berk, L.S., Noha, D. et al. (2014). 'The effect of humour on short-term memory in older adults: A new component for whole-person wellness', *Advances* 28(2), Spring.

Bains, G.S. et al. (2015). 'Humour's effect on short-term memory in healthy and diabetic older adults', *Alternative Therapies* 21(3), May/June.

Amir, O., and Biederman, I. (2016). 'The Neural Correlates of Humor Creativity', *Frontiers in Human Neuroscience* 10, 597.

Weinberg, M., Hammond, T., and Cummins, R. (2014). 'The impact of laughter yoga on subjective well-being: A pilot study', *European Journal of Humour Research* 1(4), 25–34.

Brown, S., and Vaughan, C. (2009). *Play: How it Shapes the Brain, Opens the Imagination, and Invigorates the Soul*, Avery.

Keith, M.J., Anderson, G., Gaskin, J. et al. (2018). 'Team Gaming for Team-building: Effects on Team Performance', *AIS Transactions on Human-Computer Interaction.*

Proyer, R., and Ruch, W. (2011). 'The virtuousness of adult playfulness: The relation of playfulness with strengths of character', *Psychology of Well-Being: Theory, Research and Practice* 1.

8. Mindset – dial up the positive

Diamond, D. (2015). *Beyond Resilience: Trench Tested Tools to Thrive Under Pressure*, ebook, NogginStorm.

Dweck, C. (2014). 'The power of believing that you can improve', TED talk, November.

Dweck, C. (2007). *Mindset: The New Psychology of Success*, Ballantine Books.

Part III: Thriving

9. Rest and recovery – the key to resilience

Bönstrup, M., Iturrate, I., Thompson, R. et al. (2019). 'A Rapid Form of Offline Consolidation in Skill Learning', *Current Biology* 29(8), 1348–51.

Gruber, M.J., Ritchey, M., Wang, S.-F. et al. (2016). 'Post-learning Hippocampal Dynamics Promote Preferential Retention of Rewarding Events', *Neuron* 89(5), 1110–20.

Nakano, T., Kato, M., Morito, Y. et al. (2012). 'Blink-related activation of the resting network', *Proceedings of the National Academy of Sciences*, December.

Vatansever, D., Menon, D.K., and Stamatakis, E.A. (2017). 'Default mode contributions to automated information processing', *Proceedings of the National Academy of Sciences*, November.

Vessel, E.A., Isik, A.I., Belfi, A.M. et al. (2019). 'The default-mode network represents aesthetic appeal that generalizes across visual domains', *Proceedings of the National Academy of Sciences*, September.

Marcora, S.M., Staiano, W., and Manning, V. (2009). 'Mental fatigue impairs physical performance in humans', *Journal of Applied Physiology*, March 1.

Danziger, S., Levav, J., and Avnaim-Pesso, L. (2011). 'Extraneous factors in judicial decisions', *Proceedings of the National Academy of Sciences*, April.

Coleman, J., and Coleman, J. (2012). 'The Upside of Downtime', *Harvard Business Review*, 6 December.

Ericsson, K.A. (2011). 'The Influence of Experience and Deliberate Practice on the Development of Superior Expert Performance'. *The Cambridge Handbook Of Expertise And Expert Performance*, 683–704. doi: 10.1017/cbo9780511816796.038.

De Bloom, J. (2012). 'How do vacations affect workers' health and well-being? Vacation (after-)effects and the role of vacation activities and experiences', *Academia*. BoxPress.

'The Perpetual Guardian Four-Day Week Trial', White Paper. https://4dayweek.com

'How many productive hours in a work day? Just 2 hours and 53 minutes . . .', https://www.vouchercloud.com

'Roy Morgan Leading Indicator Report: Holiday Travel Intention', https://store.roymorgan.com/

Newport, C. (2016). *Deep Work: Rules for Focused Success in a Distracted World*. Piatkus Little, Brown.

10. Sleep – not just for the wicked

Hafner, M., Stepanek, M., Taylor, J. et al. (2016). 'Why sleep matters — the economic costs of insufficient sleep: A cross-country comparative analysis', RAND Corporation, Santa Monica.

Wild, C.J., Nichols, E.S., Battista, M.E. et al. (2018). 'Dissociable effects of self-reported daily sleep duration on high-level cognitive abilities', *Sleep* 41(12), December.

Greer, S.M., Goldstein, A.N., and Walker M.P. (2013). 'The impact of sleep deprivation on food desire in the human brain', *Nature Communications* 4, 2259.

Depner, C.M. et al. (2019). 'Ad libitum weekend recovery sleep fails to prevent metabolic dysregulation during a repeating pattern of insufficient sleep and weekend recovery sleep', Current Biology 29(6), 957–67.

'Less sleep leads to more eating and more weight gain, according to new CU-Boulder study', CU Boulder Today, 11 March 2013.

Al Khatib, H., Harding, S., Darzi, J. et al. (2017). 'The effects of partial sleep deprivation on energy balance: A systematic review and meta-analysis', European Journal of Clinical Nutrition 71, 614–24.

University of Arizona Health Sciences (2018). 'Sleep loss linked to night time snacking, junk food cravings, obesity, diabetes', ScienceDaily, 1 June.

Saghir, Z., Syeda, J.N., Muhammad, A.S. et al. (2018). 'The Amygdala, Sleep Debt, Sleep Deprivation, and the Emotion of Anger: A Possible Connection?', Cureus 10(7), e2912.

Gordon, A.M., and Chen, S. (2014). 'The Role of Sleep in Interpersonal Conflict: Do Sleepless Nights Mean Worse Fights?', Social Psychological and Personality Science 5(2), 168–75.

'10 Wellness Trends for 2020', Global Wellness Institute, 28 January 2020.

Digeon, N., and Koble, A. (2011). 'Effects of Constructive Worry, Imagery Distraction, and Gratitude Interventions on Sleep Quality: A Pilot Trial', Applied Psychology Health and Wellbeing, May.

11. Food to boost your mood

Jacka, F.N., O'Neil, A., Opie, R. et al. (2017). 'A randomised controlled trial of dietary improvement for adults with major depression (the 'SMILES' trial)', BMC Medicine 15, 23.

Adan, R.A.H., van der Beek, E.H., Buitelaar, J.K. et al. (2019). 'Nutritional psychiatry: Towards improving mental health by what you eat', European Neuropsychopharmacology 29(12), 1321–32.

Dunbar, R.I.M. (2017). 'Breaking Bread: The Functions of Social Eating', Adaptive Human Behavior and Physiology 3, 198–211.

Knüppel, A., Shipley, M.J., Llewellyn, C.H. et al. (2017). 'Sugar intake from sweet food and beverages, common mental disorder and depression: Prospective findings from the Whitehall II study. Science Reports 7, 6287.

Global Council on Brain Health (2019). Brain Health and Wellness: Supplements, https://aarp.org.

Zhou, A., and Hyppönen, E. (2019). 'Long-term coffee consumption, caffeine metabolism genetics, and risk of cardiovascular disease: A prospective analysis of up to 347,077 individuals and 8368 cases', *American Journal of Clinical Nutrition* 109(3), 509–16.

Crippa, A., Discacciati, A., Larsson, S.C. et al. (2014). 'Coffee consumption and mortality from all causes, cardiovascular disease, and cancer: A dose-response meta-analysis', *American Journal of Epidemiology* 180(8), 763–75.

Loftfield, E., Cornelis, M.C., Caporaso, N. et al. (2018). 'Association of Coffee Drinking with Mortality by Genetic Variation in Caffeine Metabolism: Findings from the UK Biobank, *JAMA Internal Medicine* 178(8), 1086–97.

Yuan, S., Li, X., Jin, Y. et al. (2017). 'Chocolate Consumption and Risk of Coronary Heart Disease, Stroke, and Diabetes: A Meta-Analysis of Prospective Studies', *Nutrients* 9(7), 688.

12. Exercise as medicine

AIHW (2017). 'Risk factors to health', web report, 7 August.

Loprinzi, P.D. (2016). 'Healthy Lifestyle Characteristics and Their Joint Association with Cardiovascular Disease Biomarkers in US Adults, *Mayo Clinic Proceedings* 91(4), 432–42.

World Health Organization (2018). Physical Activity: Key facts, 23 February.

Ratey, J., and Hagerman, E. (2008). *Spark: The Revolutionary New Science of Exercise and the Brain*, Little, Brown and Company.

Ioannis, D., Morres, I.D., Hatzigeorgiadis, A., et al. (2018). 'Aerobic exercise for adult patients with major depressive disorder in mental health services: A systematic review and meta-analysis', *Depression and Anxiety*, 18 October.

Zhao, M., Veeranki, S.P., Li, S. et al. (2018). 'Beneficial associations of low and large doses of leisure time physical activity with all-cause, cardiovascular disease and cancer mortality: A national cohort study of 88,140 US adults', *British Journal of Sports Medicine* 53(22).

Merghani, A., Malhotra, A., and Sharma, S. (2016). 'The U-shaped relationship between exercise and cardiac morbidity', *Trends in Cardiovascular Medicine* 26(3), 232–40.

Erickson, K.I., Voss, M.W., Prakash, R.S. et al. (2011). 'Exercise training increases size of hippocampus and improves memory', *Proceedings of the National Academy of Sciences* 108(7), 3017–22.

Godman, H. (2014). 'Regular exercise changes the brain to improve memory, thinking skills', Harvard Health Blog, Harvard Medical School, April 9.

Schuch, F.B., Vancampfort, D., Firth, J. et al. (2018). 'Physical Activity and Incident Depression: A Meta-Analysis of Prospective Cohort Studies', *American Journal of Psychiatry* 175(7), 631–48.

Chekroud, S.R., Gueorguieva, R., Zheutlin, A.B. et al. (2018). 'Association between physical exercise and mental health in 1.2 million individuals in the USA between 2011 and 2015: A cross-sectional study', *The Lancet Psychiatry* 5(9), 739–48.

Sibold, J.S., and Berg, K.M. (2010). 'Mood enhancement persists for up to 12 hours following aerobic exercise: A pilot study', *Percept. Mot. Skills* 111(2), 333–42.

De Cocker, K., Bourdeaudhuij, I., Brown, W. et al. (2010). 'The pedometer-based community intervention "10,000 Steps Ghent": Who used a pedometer and who increased their steps?', *Journal of Science and Medicine in Sport* 12.

Ding, D., Lawson, K.D., Kolbe-Alexander, T.L. et al. (2016). 'The economic burden of physical inactivity: A global analysis of major non-communicable diseases', *The Lancet* 388(10051), 1311–24.

Lee, I.-M., Shiroma, E.J., Lobelo, F. et al. (2012). 'Effect of physical inactivity on major non-communicable diseases worldwide: An analysis of burden of disease and life expectancy', *The Lancet*, 18 July. www.getbritainstanding.org

Buckley, J.P., Hedge, A., Yates, T. et al. (2015). 'The sedentary office', *British Journal of Sports Medicine* 49(21), 1–6.

Finch, L.E., Tomiyama, A.J., and Ward, A. (2017). 'Taking a Stand: The Effects of Standing Desks on Task Performance and Engagement', *Int. J. Environ. Res. Public Health* 14(8), 939.

13. Music and dance

Collins, A.M. (2018). 'Dancing, Mindfulness, and Our Emotions: Embracing the Mind, Body, and Sole', MA thesis, Cuny Academic Works.

Rehfeld, K., Müller, P., Aye, N. et al. (2017). 'Dancing or Fitness Sport? The Effects of Two Training Programs on Hippocampal Plasticity and Balance Abilities in Healthy Seniors', *Frontiers in Human Neuroscience*, 15 June.

Powers, R. (2010). 'Use It or Lose It: Dancing Makes You Smarter', 30 July, socialdance.stanford.edu

Aalbers, S., Fusar-Poli, L., Freeman, R.E. et al. (2017). 'Music Therapy for Depression', *Frontiers in Human Neuroscience*, 16 November, p. 305.

Trappe, H.J., and Voit, G. (2016). 'The Cardiovascular Effect of Musical Genres: A randomized controlled study on the effect of compositions by W. A. Mozart, J. Strauss, and ABBA', *Dtsch Arztebl Int* 113, 347–52.

Levitin, D. (2019). *This Is Your Brain on Music*, Penguin.

Cooper, L. (2019). 'Using Music as Medicine — finding the optimum music listening 'dosage'. Deezer Health and Wellbeing Research, www.britishacademyofsoundtherapy.com

National Institutes of Health (2019). 'NIH awards $20 million over five years to bring together music therapy and music science', US Department of Health and Human Services, 19 September.

Goel, S. (2016). 'Listening to music makes you a better employee', grapevineonline, 13 June.

Mindlin, G., DuRousseau, D., and Cardillo, J. (2012). *Your Playlist Can Change Your Life: 10 Proven Ways Your Favorite Music Can Revolutionize Your Health, Memory, Organization, Alertness and More*, Sourcebooks.

14. Blue and green – complete the scene

Selhub, E.M., and Logan, A. (2012). *Your Brain on Nature: The Science of Nature's Influence on Your Health Happiness and Vitality*, Wiley Canada.

Klepeis, N.E., Nelson, W.C., Ott, W.R. et al. The National Human Activity Pattern Survey (NHAPS): A resource for assessing exposure to environmental pollutants.

Global Wellness Summit (2019). Joining Together. Shaping the Future, www.globalbwellnesssummit.com

White, M.P., Alcock, I., Grellier, J. et al. (2019). 'Spending at least 120 minutes a week in nature is associated with good health and wellbeing', *Scientific Reports* 9(1).

Berman, M.G., Kross, E., Krpan, K.M. et al. (2012). 'Interacting with nature improves cognition and affect for individuals with depression', *Journal of Affective Disorders*.

Pasanen, T.P., White, M.P., Wheeler, B.W. et al. (2019). 'Neighbourhood blue space, health and wellbeing: The mediating role of different types of physical activity', *Environment International* 131.

Hansen, M.M., Jones, R., and Tocchini, K. (2017). 'Shinrin-Yoku (Forest Bathing) and Nature Therapy: A State-of-the-Art Review', *International Journal of Environmental Research and Public Health* 14(8), 851.

Allen, S. (2018). 'The Science of Awe', white paper, Greater Good Science Center, UC Berkeley.

Li, Q. (2010). 'Effect of forest bathing trips on human immune function', *Environmental Health and Preventive Medicine* 15(1), 9–17.

Nicholls, W.J. (2015). *Blue Mind: The remarkable effects of water on our health and wellbeing*, Bay Back Books.

Blue Health Project: https://bluehealth2020.eu

Gregory N. Bratman, G.N., Hamilton, J.P., Hahn, K.S. et al. (2015). 'Nature reduces rumination and sgPFC activation', *Proceedings of the National Academy of Sciences* 112(28), 8567–72.

James, P., Hart, J.E., Banay, R.F., and Laden, F. (2016). 'Exposure to Greenness and Mortality in a Nationwide Prospective Cohort Study of Women', *Environmental Health Perspectives* 124(9), 1344–52.

United Technologies (2020). 'The impact of green buildings on cognitive function', The Buildingomics COGfx Study.

Stringer, L. (2019). *The Healthy Workplace: How to Improve the Well being of Your Employees — and Boost Your Company's Bottom Line*, Amacom.

University of Exeter (2014). 'Why plants in the office make us more productive', *ScienceDaily*, 1 September.

Nieuwenhuis, M., Knight, C., Postmes, T., and Haslam, S.A. (2014). 'The Relative Benefits of Green Versus Lean Office Space: Three Field Experiments', *Journal of Experimental Psychology: Applied* 20(3). 28 July. Advance online publication.

Atchley, R.A., Strayer, D.L., and Atchley P. (2012). 'Creativity in the Wild: Improving Creative Reasoning through Immersion in Natural Settings', *PLOS One*, 12 December.

Barton, J., and Pretty, J. (2010). 'What Is the Best Dose of Nature and Green Exercise for Improving Mental Health? A Multi-Study Analysis', *Environmental Science and Technology* 44(10), 3947–55.

Part IV: Human

Lieberman, M. (2013). *Social: Why Our Brains Are Hard Wired to Connect*, Crown Publishers, New York.

Meyer, M.L. Davachi, L., Ochsner, K.N., and Lieberman, M.D. (2018). 'Evidence that Default Network Connectivity During Rest Consolidates Social Information', *Cerebral Cortex*.

Schmälzle, R., O'Donnell, M.B., Garcia, J.O. et al. (2017). 'Brain connectivity dynamics during social interaction reflect social network structure', *Proceedings of the National Academy of Sciences*.

Eisenberger, N.I., Lieberman, M.D., and Williams, K.D. (2003). 'Does rejection hurt? An FMRI study of social exclusion', *Science* 302(5643), 290–2.

15. Trust and respect

www.edelman.com/trustbarometer

Barefoot, J.C., Maynard, K.E., Beckham, J.C. et al. (1998). 'Trust, health, and longevity', *Journal of Behavioural Medicine* 21(6), 517–26.

Holt-Lunstad, J., Smith, T.B., and Layton, J.B. (2010). 'Social Relationships and Mortality Risk: A Meta-analytic Review', *PLoS Med* 7(7).

House, J.S., Landis, K.R., and Umberson, D. (1998). Social relationships and health, *Science* 241(4865), 540–5.

Huppert, F.A., Clark, A., Marks, N., and Siegrist, J. (2008). 'Measuring Well-being Across Europe: Description of the ESS Well-being Module and Preliminary Findings', *Social Indicators Research* 91(3).

Wei, D., Lee, D., Cox, C.D. et al. (2015). 'Endocannabinoid signaling mediates oxytocin-driven social reward', *PNAS*, 26 October.

Kirsch, L.P., Krahé, C, Blom, N. et al. (2017). 'Reading the mind in the touch: Neurophysiological specificity in the communication of emotions by touch', *Neuropsychologia* 116, *Part A*, 136–49.

Zak, P. (2018). *The Trust Factor*, HarperCollins Focus US.

Brown, B. (2017). *Rising Strong: How the ability to reset transforms the way we live, love, parent and lead*. Penguin Random House.

Edmondson, A. (2018). *The Fearless Organisation: Creating Psychological Safety in the Workplace for Learning, Innovation and Growth*, Wiley.

Snyder, R.A. (2016). *The Social Cognitive Neuroscience of Leading Organisational Change*, Routledge.

16. Kindness and compassion

Darley, J.M., and Batson, C.D., (1973). ' "From Jerusalem to Jericho": A Study of Situational and Dispositional Variables in Helping Behavior', *Journal of Personality and Social Psychology*, 27, 100–8.

Rowland, L., and Curry, O.S. (2019). 'A range of kindness activities boost happiness', *Journal of Social Psychology* 159(3), 340–3.

Nelson, S.K., Layous, K., Cole, S.W., and Lyubomirsky, S. (2016). 'Do unto others or treat yourself? The effects of prosocial and self-focused behavior on psychological flourishing', *Emotion* 16(6), 850–61.

Dutton, J.E., Workman, K.M., and Hardin, A.E. (2014). 'Compassion at work', SHA School, Cornell University.

Trzeciak, S., and Mazzarelli, A. (2019). *Compassionomics: The Revolutionary Scientific Evidence that Caring Makes a Difference*, Studer Group.

Dr Kristin Neff, https://self-compassion.org/

17. Empathy: 'I feel your pain'

Rizzolatti, G., and Craighero, L. (2004). 'The Mirror-Neuron System', *Annual Review of Neuroscience* 27, 169–92.

Riess, H. (2018). *The Empathy Effect: Seven Neuroscience-Based Keys for Transforming the Way We Live, Love, Work and Connect Across Differences*, Sounds True Colorado.

Decety J., and Fotopoulou, A. (2015). 'Why empathy has a beneficial impact on others in medicine: Unifying theories', *Frontiers in Behavioral Neuroscience* 8, 457.

2019 State of Workplace Empathy, www.businesssolver.com.

Conclusion

Clear, J. (2018). *Atomic Habits: Tiny Changes, Remarkable Results*, Random House.

Index

adaptability 4, 23, 27, 69, 97,
    110, 115, 160, 260
adenosine 125, 148
adrenaline 11
alcohol consumption 13,
    16, 139, 143, 159, 165,
    167–168, 228
    limits 167–168
    sleep, effect on 148–149
Alzheimer's disease 178, 232
amygdala 15, 68, 72, 141
anterior cingulate cortex 125
anterior cingulate gyrus 15
anterior insula 69
anterior temporal cortex 51
anxiety 2, 7–8, 9, 15, 22, 36,
    52, 53, 75, 93, 105, 108–
    109, 122, 141, 142, 149,
    154, 181, 221, 248, 249
    exercise 175, 179, 181
    laughter and 89
    music 197, 199, 200
    nature of 7–8

treatment 35, 53, 65, 73, 74,
    80, 83, 89, 95, 109, 168, 179,
    199, 207, 209, 241
atherosclerosis 136
attention 66, 68, 69, 71, 72,
    122, 124, 127, 138, 139,
    150–151, 179, 204, 210–
    212; see also cognition
auditory cortex 196

balance, physical 185, 187,
    188, 194
barn raising 237
blame 3, 100, 101
blood pressure 52, 61, 73, 80,
    88, 89, 123, 149, 168, 182,
    196, 198, 207, 228
blood vessels 168
Blue Zones 34, 154–155;
    see also diet
brain 51, 60, 68, 69, 15, 69–70,
    71–72, 73, 89–90, 93,
    120–121, 125, 141, 178, 180,

193–194, 195, 196, 209, 226;
see also entries under the
names of parts of the brain
brown-out 11–12
burnout 4, 6, 10, 12–16, 26,
35, 68, 93, 99, 121, 249,
256; *see also* overwhelm;
overwork; stress
effects on brain 14–16
features 12–13
bushfires 2019–20,
Australian 102–103
Busy Brain Syndrome *see also*
negativity; overthinking;
rumination; worrying
breaks, taking 144–145
defined 144
journaling 145, 146
planning ahead 145–146

caffeine 148, 149, 166, 169;
see also coffee
cardiovascular function/
disease 41, 52, 62, 88,
136–137; *see also* heart
attack; heart disease
and health
cerebellum 196
chocolate 34, 165, 168–169
cholesterol 33, 62, 87, 88, 169
coffee 125, 144, 148, 165,
166–167, 201, 237, 246,
256; *see also* caffeine
cognition and cognitive load
14, 60, 70, 68, 93, 121,
121, 122, 126, 136, 139,

149, 150, 168, 175, 178,
180, 184, 187, 193–194,
199, 206, 255; *see also*
attention; learning ability;
memory and recall
exercise and 177–178
nature and 209–210, 211
purpose and 41–42
sleep and 139–140
cognitive behavioural therapy
(CBT-i) 151
cognitive therapy 73
colouring in activity 81
comfort zone 110–
111, 186–187
compassion, defined 257;
see also kindness and
compassion
connection, social 216–219;
see also disconnection;
empathy; kindness and
compassion; loneliness;
respect; social pain;
thriving; trust
benefits of 217–219
case study 223
creating 95–96
empathy 253–261
food and 157–158, 166–167
importance 222
increasing 237, 256
kindness and compassion
243–251
loneliness 21–222
need for 216–217
reconnecting 25–29

respect 238–241
social media 220–221
social pain 17–18, 218–220
trust 225–237
wellbeing and 16–19,
    219, 247–249
work 237
conscious awareness 80
cortisol 11, 41, 68, 74, 86, 88,
    137, 141, 148, 169, 181,
    196, 206, 248
creativity and creative
    thinking 2, 25, 27, 35, 43,
    81, 90, 93, 94, 96, 121, 127,
    150, 192, 193, 195, 196,
    198, 200, 209, 210, 212
current issues 2, 3–23;
    see also anxiety; burnout;
    depression; disconnection;
    fatigue; loneliness;
    overwhelm; overwork;
    stress; wellbeing
    anxiety 2, 7–8
    burnout 6, 12–16
    depression 2, 9
    disconnection 16, 19–23
    exhaustion 4
    fatigue 5–6
    loneliness 2, 6, 16–23
    overwhelm 2, 4, 7, 26
    overwork 6, 10–12, 13
    stress 6, 11, 12, 14–15, 16,
        17, 18, 19
    trip hazards 7
    wellbeing, lack of 6–9
Cyberball 220

dance 28, 191–195;
    see also music
age 193–194
benefits 193–194, 195
building skills 201–202
emotions 192
mindfulness 192–193
movement therapy 192–195
work, at 195
death see disease; mortality
decision making 2, 12, 22,
    71, 78, 96, 106, 122,
    125, 138, 141, 144, 175,
    225, 226, 229
default mode network
    (DMN) 120–121
dementia 166, 180, 197
depression 2, 3, 6, 22, 52, 75,
    93, 125, 142, 149, 181, 248
    causes 22, 169, 209
    diet 155–156
    exercise 175, 179, 181
    indicators 9
    management 73–74
    mindfulness 73–74
    music 197, 199
    treatment 35, 53, 65, 73,
        74, 75–76, 91, 155–
        156, 168, 207
diabetes 21, 137, 138, 169, 180,
    182, 184, 206
diet 28, 114, 153–171; see also
    alcohol; caffeine; chocolate;
    coffee; supplements
    Blue Zones 34, 154–155
    brain effects 155, 168

building skills 170–171
changing 157, 163–164
connection, social
    155, 157–158
depression 155–156
emotions 159–160
longevity 154
mental health 155–157
microbiome 160–164
Modified Mediterranean
    Diet 155–156
mood-boosting 153–171
obstacles to good 158–160
pre- and probiotics 162
risks of poor 169–170
sleep and 137–138
Standard
    Australian Diet 156
sugar 156, 159
takeaway foods 157, 158
thriving 28, 114
wine 165, 167–168
difference,
    acknowledging 238–239
digital detox 123–124
disconnection, social 6,
    16–23, 26; *see also*
    connection; loneliness;
    social pain
causes 19–21
effects 22–23
resolving 23
social pain 218–219
disease *see* Alzheimer's
    disease; anxiety; blood
    pressure; Busy Brain

Syndrome; cardiovascular
    function/disease;
    dementia; depression;
    diabetes; disconnection;
    heart attack; heart disease
    and health; inflammation;
    loneliness; obesity;
    overwork; rumination;
    social pain; stress; stroke;
    wellbeing; wellbeing,
    mental; worrying
dopamine 59, 51, 89, 196

eating *see* diet
ecotherapy 207
emotions, management
    of 76, 91, 141, 192,
    193, 194; *see also*
    anxiety; connection;
    disconnection; depression;
    empathy; happiness;
    loneliness; mood;
    negativity; optimism;
    positivity; social pain
diet 159–160
mindfulness and 71–76
empathy 28–29, 61, 253–261
benefits of 256–257
brain effects 225
building 257–260
building skills 261
case study 254
components 255
curiosity 258
defined 253, 260
eye contact 257

honesty 260
judgement,
    avoiding 258–259
    language tone 259
    listening 258
endocrine system 69, 87, 133
endorphins 87, 89, 91,
    164, 178, 198
epinephrine 88
exclusion 17–18; *see also*
    disconnection; social pain
exercise 28, 114, 173–189;
    see also dance; music
    amount needed 181–183
    attitudes to 173, 175
    benefits of 174–177
    brain benefits 177–181
    building skills 188–189
    cognition 177–178
    fatigue 176–177
    goals, fitness 186–187
    happiness 174, 179–181
    high-intensity interval
        training 186–187
    longevity 178
    memory 178–179
    mental wellbeing 178
    opportunities for 187–188
    routine 181
    sitting, danger of 183–188
    10,000 steps 182–183
    walking 174

fatigue 5–6, 176–177; *see also*
    overwhelm; overwork;
    rest and recovery; stress

mental 210–211
    story 131–132
focus, outward 58
food *see* diet
friends and friendship 16–17;
    see also connection;
    disconnection; loneliness;
    social pain
    exclusion 17–18
    work 18–19

gamma waves 69, 89–90
generosity 58–59; *see also*
    gratitude; kindness
ghrelin 137
gratitude 27, 49–56
    benefits 50–53
    brain effects 51–53
    building skills 56
    compassion 49, 68
    cultivating attitude 53–55
    happiness and 50–53, 55
    journaling 49–50, 52–53,
        54, 146
    journaling story 49–50
    lack of 53
    recognition story 54–55
    stress hormones 52
green certified offices 211
grey matter 51, 68, 70

happiness *see also* connection;
    emotions; gratitude;
    helping others; kindness
    and compassion; laughter;
    mindset; mindfulness;

play; purpose
and meaning
benefits 35
building 38
causes 32–33
exercise and 174, 179–181
gratitude and 50–53, 55
health and
relationships and 33–34
importance 37–38
improving 37, 94
ingredients of 27, 31–111
lack of 2, 36
laughter and 90–91
purpose and 42–43
resilience 35
transience of 36
trust and 227
work, at 37
health and wellbeing
see disease; immune
system; inflammation;
longevity; mortality;
wellbeing;
wellbeing, mental
helping others 27, 57–64
brain effects 59–63
building skills 64
happy hormones 59
health effect 61–63
stress reduction 60–61
time poverty effects 63
volunteering story 57–58
heart attack 11, 41, 136, 137,
184, 166, 169, 256; see also
cardiovascular function/

disease; heart disease
and health
heart disease and health
14, 21, 35, 137, 180,
184, 198, 206; see also
cardiovascular function/
disease; heart attack
hippocampus 69, 178, 193–194
hoarding 107
hormones see also adrenaline;
cortisol; dopamine;
endorphins; epinephrine;
ghrelin; hypocretin; leptin;
melatonin; noradrenaline;
oxytocin; serotonin;
thyroid stimulating
hormone; testosterone;
vasopressin
feel good 180
happy 59
sleep 133, 137
stress 11, 15, 52, 88, 89, 148,
149, 181, 196, 206, 248
human, being see also
kindness and compassion;
empathy; respect; trust
building skills 224
components 28–29,
215–260
empathy 253–261
kindness and
compassion 243–251
nature of 28–29
summary 215–224
trust and respect 225–242
hypocretin 137

imagination *see* creativity
immune system 22, 69, 198
  boosting 35, 41, 52,
    86–87, 88, 89, 161, 199,
    206, 207, 248
impostor syndrome 8, 74,
  75, 110, 250
inflammation 35, 42, 52, 62,
  68, 74, 87, 136, 156, 159,
  161, 166, 248
insomnia 140
irrational, predictably 2

job security 4, 8, 11,
  87, 226, 228
Jymmin 197

kindness and compassion
  28–29, 68, 243–251
  benefits of 247–249
  building skills 251
  conscious seeking 244–245
  cultivating 249
  fallibility 250–251
  happiness 245–246
  humanity 247–251
  mindfulness 251
  motivation for 244–245
  self-compassion 249–250
  self-forgiveness 250–251
  wellbeing 247–249

laughter 27, 85–93, 93–98;
  see also play
  anxiety 89
  building skills 97–98

  creativity 90
  happiness 90–91
  health benefits 86–93
  heart health 87
  immunity 86–87
  increasing 91–93
  longevity 88
  macabre 86
  memory 89–90, 93
  stress reduction 85, 88–89
Laughercise© 88
learning ability 2, 68, 89–90,
  93, 120, 166, 178, 180, 194,
  196, 216; *see also* memory
leptin 137
limbic system 15,
  52, 71–72, 76
loneliness 2, 6, 16–23, 26, 228;
  see also disconnection;
  social pain
  effects 22
  social isolation 21–22
longevity 22, 68, 88,
  178; *see also* Blue
  Zones; mortality
  diet 154
  exercise 178
  laughter 88
  nature and 209–210
  purpose and
    meaning 40–41
  trust 227–228

Maslach Burnout Inventory 16
MBSR course 76
meditation *see* mindfulness

melatonin 80, 134, 143, 147, 150
memory and recall 15, 41–42, 68, 69, 71, 89, 90, 93, 120, 133, 139, 148–149, 159, 168, 169, 178–179, 180, 181, 194, 196–197, 210, 231
microbiome 154, 160–164, 169
mindfulness 27, 65–83
  app 80
  benefits 67
  brain effects 67–70
  breathing 72–73
  building skills 83
  case study 75–76
  decision-making 71
  emotional control 71–76
  explained 66
  meditation 65, 72
  method 76–81
  moments, benefits of mindful 81–83
  sleep 149–150
  sleep vs 80–81
  stress 65, 73–74
  useful, management of 76–77
  work at 79–80
mindset 27, 99–111; see also imposter syndrome
  building skills 111
  bushfires examples 102–103
  changing your 106–111
  choice of 104–105
  comfort zone 110–111
  goals 111
  growth vs fixed 104, 105
  intention 108
  negative self-talk 107
  negativity 105–106, 108–109
  noise, reducing 108
  perfectionism 109–110
  positivity 110
  shifting 101
  stress, dealing with 105–106
  thoughts, managing 106–107
  thriver 102–104
  ties of the past 101
  victim vs survivor story 99–100, 103
  victimhood vs survivorhood vs thriving 100–102, 110
mood 60, 63, 88, 89, 106–107, 168, 192, 198, 210, 236; see also anxiety; connection; depression; disconnection; emotions; exclusion; loneliness; social pain
  boosting 23, 35, 50, 51, 53, 59, 61, 68, 88, 89, 91, 92, 94, 95, 97, 133, 139, 227, 245
  diet 153–171
  disorders 6, 9, 10, 71, 74, 149, 159, 181, 198, 256
  exercise 178, 180, 181, 206
  mindset and 192, 198, 199
  music and dance 195, 197, 199, 201
  nature 204, 206, 207, 212

mortality 10, 11, 40, 86,
    88, 102, 137, 156, 179,
    183, 206, 208, 210, 228;
    see also disease
Move It Monday 195
music 28, 115, 195–201;
    see also dance
    ambient noise 198
    brain effect 196–198
    building skills 201–202
    connection 198–199
    creativity 200
    memory 196–197
    mental wellbeing 197–198
    mood 192, 198, 199
    pain 197
    singing 197, 198–199
    stress 199
    wellbeing 198
    work, at 199–200, 201
myopia 206

nature 28, 115, 203–213
    attention 210–212
    brain benefits 205–212
    building skills 213
    calming effects 207–208
    deficit 204–205
    greenery 210, 211, 212
    mental fatigue 210–211
    mood 210
    rumination 209
    swimming 209
    wind 207
    work 210–211
negative loop 37

negativity 12, 54, 71–72, 74,
    105–106, 107, 141–142;
    see also worrying
    bias 141
    dealing with 15, 36
    mindfulness and
        76, 105–106,
        108–109
    reducing 51, 52, 61, 91, 92,
        94–96, 237, 248
    self-talk 74, 100, 107, 110
    stewing 37–38, 141–142
neural circuits 51, 69–70,
    105, 197, 270
neural connectivity 195
neural pathways 196, 219, 269
neural patterns 54
neural synchrony 231
neurobiology 269
neurochemicals 178
neurogenesis 180
neuroinflammation 159
neurons 51, 140, 255
neuroplasticity 15, 69, 74, 93,
    95, 180, 194, 195
neuroprotection 166
neurotransmitters
    125, 161, 168
noradrenaline 73
nutrition *see* diet

obesity and weight
    management 136, 137,
    138, 151, 153, 169, 181,
    198, 206, 228, 232
    sleep and 137–138

optimism 35, 52, 54, 107, 110, 114, 248
overthinking 4, 5, 78, 125, 144; *see also* Busy Brain Syndrome; negativity; rumination; worrying
overwhelm 2, 4, 7, 13, 16, 17, 26, 63, 70, 83, 93, 102, 110, 208, 244, 267; *see also* burnout; overwork; stress
overwork 6, 10–12, 13–14, 17, 18, 23, 26, 37, 101, 122; *see also* burnout; rest and recovery; stress
  heath risks 11–12
oxytocin 34, 59, 198, 217, 227, 229–230, 232, 233, 234
OzHarvest 62

pain management 52, 68, 76, 197
panic buying 109
parasympathetic nervous system 73
passive aggression 221–222
perfectionism 74, 75–76
  avoiding 109–110
play 27, 93–98; *see also* laughter
  brain benefits 93–97
  building skills 97–98
  connection and 95–96
  creativity 96
  decision making 96
  power of 93–97

productivity 97
  work improvement 96
polyphenols 168
positive feedback loop 35
positivity 19, 27, 32, 36, 42, 53, 70, 86–87, 90, 106, 107, 139, 194, 222; *see also* emotions; happiness; mindset; negativity; optimism
  increasing 38, 50, 51, 54, 59, 69, 91, 92, 110, 146, 154, 169, 245, 272
prefrontal cortex (PFC) 15, 69, 70, 71, 72, 125, 141, 179, 196, 209
present, being 206–207
productivity vs humanity 115
psychoneuroimmunology (PNI) 87
purpose and meaning 27, 39–47
  achieving 43–47
  brain benefits 40–43
  building 47
  cognition 41–42
  genetics 42
  goals, setting 45–46
  happiness 42–43
  health and wellbeing 41
  longevity 40–41
  sleep 41
  story of loss of 40

recall *see* memory and recall
reconnecting 25–29; *see also* connection; disconnection

rejection *see* disconnection;
   social pain
relationships and 33–34,
   142; *see also* connection;
   disconnection; negativity;
   positivity; reconnecting;
   respect; social pain; trust
   forming 229–230
   health and 33–34
   importance of 228
resilience 67, 117–127; *see also*
   rest and recovery
   boosting 118, 119
   happiness and 35
   workshop story 117–119
respect and 28–29, 238–241;
   see also trust
   building skills 240–241
   difference,
      acknowledging 238–239
   interest, showing 240–241
   mutual 238–241
   names, knowing 240
   presence, acknowledging
      239–240
rest and recovery 27, 114,
   117–129; *see also* exercise;
   overwhelm; overwork;
   resilience; work hours
   brain benefits 119–121
   breaks, benefits of 120–123,
      144–145
   building skills 129
   cognitive load management
      (CM) 121–123
   holidays 128

mental fatigue 124–128
performance,
   improved 119–120
practice, deliberate 121
rest, types of 126–128
switching off 118
technology breaks 123–124
rumination (endless
   worrying) 53, 209;
   see also Busy Brain
   Syndrome; negativity;
   overthinking; worrying

safety 7, 16, 105–106, 111,
   217, 226, 230, 235
Screen-Free Week 123–124
self-absorption 244
self-acceptance 229, 250
self-awareness 50, 66, 102
self-belief 198, 229
self-beliefs, limiting
   100, 101, 198
self-care 5, 101, 114, 176
self-compassion 92, 250–251
self-confidence 229
self-criticism 141, 251, 260
self-doubt 5, 110
self-encouragement 107
self-esteem 50, 51, 58, 75, 221
self-image 239
self-obsession 60
self-reflection 120
self-regulation 248
self-talk, negative 74, 94,
   100, 107, 110
self-trust 228–229

self-worth 74, 212
serotonin 51, 59, 80, 148, 150,
    161, 178, 206
shrinkage, brain 70, 180
Silver Swans Ballet
    Classes 193
Singing for the Brain 197
sitting, danger of 183–188
    reducing 184–185
sleep 27, 114, 131–152; see also
    Busy Brain Syndrome; rest
    and recovery
    adenosine 125
    alcohol 148–149
    amount needed 134, 135,
        136–137, 138, 139, 150
    apnoea 140, 149, 151
    benefits of 139
    brain activity, managing
        143–152
    breathing 150
    breaks, taking 144–145
    building skills 152
    caffeine 148
    circadian rhythms 134
    cognitive effects 139–140
    disruption/deprivation
        15, 53, 125, 133,
        136–140, 151
    driving 140
    environment 146–147
    excess 136
    exercise 148, 181
    foods 148–149, 150
    genetics 136
    hormones 133, 137

improving 52–53,
    68, 144–151
jetlag 142–143
lack of 21
light 146–147
meditation vs 80–81
meditation practice
    149–150
melatonin 80, 134,
    143, 147, 150
microsleeps 140
naps 134, 150–151
need for 133
negativity 141–143
night owls 135
reducing 135, 136–137
regulation and patterns
    133–135, 144
relationships 142
rituals 146
secrets of 133–140
smoking 149
story, fatigue 131–132
technology 147–148
timing 134–135
weekend catchup 138
weight and 137–138
worry 141
SMILES Trial 155–156
smoking, health effects of 22,
    149, 156, 183, 228
social contagion 109
social media, effects of 20,
    220–221
social pain 218–220; see also
    disconnection

causes 219, 235
effects 219–220
stress 4, 5, 6, 7–8, 10, 12,
    14–15, 16, 17, 26, 35, 35,
    36, 63, 71, 87, 91, 105, 109,
    119, 121, 127, 154, 159,
    174, 210, 245, ; *see also*
    burnout; overwork
brain effects 14–16, 71–72
effects of 37, 76, 87, 108, 115,
hormones 11, 15, 52,
    88, 89, 148, 149, 181,
    196, 206, 248
managing 18, 41, 43, 50,
    51, 52, 53, 54, 60–61, 65,
    66, 67, 68, 69, 71, 73–74,
    75–76, 88–89, 90, 91,
    93, 94, 95, 98, 123, 127,
    138, 145, 150, 157, 159,
    174, 179–180, 185, 195,
    199, 205, 207, 208, 209,
    212, 226, 227, 233, 248,
    249, 256, 265
mindfulness and 76–83
safe place and 105–106
story 137–138
stroke 11, 14, 41, 136, 169, 180,
    180, 182
supplements 164–165
Suprachiasmatic Nucleus
    (SCN) 134

testosterone 137
thought *see* cognition
thriving 113–213
    choice for 23

defined 114
diet 28, 114, 153–171
exercise 28, 114, 173–189
music and dance 28, 114,
    191–202
nature, time in 28,
    114, 203–213
requirements 27–28
rest and recovery 27, 114,
    117–129
sleep 27, 114, 131–152
summary 114–115
thyroid stimulating
    hormone 137
tiredness *see* fatigue; rest and
    recovery; sleep
toilet paper panic 109
triglycerides 169
trust and 28–29, 225–237;
    see also respect
    brain effects 226, 227–228
    building skills 240–241
    case studies 235, 236
    community, building 237
    diminishing 226–227, 227
    eye contact 231
    happiness 227
    hugging 232–234
    importance 226
    instinct 230–231
    lack of 236
    longevity 227–228
    loss of 234, 235
    nurturing 229–230
    resilience 228
    safety 226, 230, 235

self- 228–229
story, importance of 225
touch 232–234
wellbeing 227–228
work, at 234–236

ultradian rhythm 144

vagus nerve 73, 232
vasopressin 59
victim vs survivor story
99–100, 103
victimhood vs survivorhood
vs thriving 100–102, 110
volunteering
see helping others

wellbeing 178; *see also*
diet; disease; exercise;
longevity; microbiome;
wellbeing, mental
connection and 16–19, 219
environment and 203–204
essentials 26, 27
improving 67, 68, 180
kindness 247–249
learned skill 60
music 198
nature 205–206
purpose and meaning 41
risks to 4
trust 227–228
wellbeing, mental 108; *see also*
connection; disease;

emotions; relationships;
rest and recovery
connection and 16–19
exercise 178
improving 50–51, 67, 68, 93,
119, 192–193
kindness 247–249
lack of 6–9
learned skill 60
music in 197–198
nature 205
wine 165, 167–168;
see also alcohol
With One Voice choirs 198
work, attitudes to 18–19,
13–14; *see also*
work hours
workaholism 13–14
work hours 10, 11, 20, 21, 63,
70, 76, 118, 123, 131, 134,
160, 176, 265; *see also*
overwhelm; overwork; rest
and recovery
worrying 8, 53, 87, 95, 105,
70–72, 141–142; *see also*
anxiety; Busy Brain
Syndrome; negativity;
overthinking; rumination

yoga 28, 193,
laughter 90–91
nidra 149
yogic breathing 73